Ratings for more than a thousand food entries using
the revolutionary Cholesterol-Saturated Fat Index,
plus a plan to keep your cholesterol in check

The Only Cholesterol Guide You'll Ever Need

One number
tells you
everything to
help you:

- lower your blood
  cholesterol level
- reduce your risk
  for heart disease
- achieve a desirable
  body weight

Joel M. Berns, D.M.D., with
Kenneth L. Cohen, M.D., F.A.C.P.
and Betsy A. Taylor, M.S., R.D.

Ⓑ Ballantine/Health/38133 (Canada $5.99) U.S. $4.99

**Look for these informative books
about your health!**

ARE YOU AT RISK?
How to Identify and Reduce Your Risk
for More Than 100 Diseases and Medical Conditions
by Carol Ann Rinzler

AT-A-GLANCE NUTRITION COUNTER
by Patricia Hausman

HOW TO CONTROL HIGH BLOOD PRESSURE
WITHOUT DRUGS
by Robert L. Rowan, M.D.

NUTRITION PRESCRIPTION
by Dr. Brian L. G. Morgan

EAN
9 780345 381330

ISBN 0-345-38133-5

50499

LOWER YOUR CHOLESTEROL AND FAT AND STILL ENJOY GREAT FOOD!

Here's just one example of a low-CSI day:

Breakfast
Fruit (any kind)
French toast, made with corn oil, no egg, and skim
  milk
Canadian bacon
Coffee with 2% milk

Lunch
Black bean soup
Turkey (white meat) on French bread with low-fat
  mayonnaise, lettuce, and tomato
Fruit (any kind)

Dinner
Manhattan clam chowder
Beef (eye of round), broiled
Baked sweet potato with margarine (corn oil)
Steamed spinach with lemon
Nonfat frozen yogurt

FOR GOOD HEALTH AND GOOD EATING, THIS IS THE ONLY CHOLESTEROL GUIDE YOU'LL EVER NEED

THE ONLY CHOLESTEROL GUIDE YOU'LL EVER NEED

Joel Berns, D.M.D.,
with Kenneth L. Cohen, M.D., F.A.C.P.
and Betsy A. Taylor, M.S., R.D.

BALLANTINE BOOKS • NEW YORK

Copyright © 1993 by Explanatory Publications, Inc.

The information in this book is based on general principles of good health and is consistent with the best medical and dietary information currently available. Neither the author, his consultants, nor the publisher intend this book to be a professional health service. Individuals looking for expert advice for themselves or family members should consult a competent health professional.

ISBN 0-345-38133-5

Manufactured in the United States of America

First Edition: January 1994

TABLE OF CONTENTS

In Gratitude

Dr. Jonathan L. Isaacsohn, former director of the Preventive Cardiology Program of the Yale University Medical School, gave initial encouragement that set this project in motion and, in its early stages, made critical comments of great importance.

Twenty-nine clinical dietitians around the country candidly reviewed the manuscript and made it more useful to their profession. Two dozen volunteer lay reviewers critiqued the work in progress to make it easier for anyone to use.

My wife, Marie Antoinette Berns, is responsible for a more readable text.

Kenneth Cohen, M.D., and Betsy Taylor, M.S., R.D., joined the work in progress. Their many hours of toil were of major importance in shaping this work.

I am most grateful to all these people whose generous help made this guide possible.

JOEL M. BERNS, D.M.D.

Preface

The higher your blood cholesterol level, the greater your risk of dying from a heart attack. This established fact is hardly news to anyone, and surely there's no shortage of information about the important influence of your diet on your blood cholesterol level. Bookstore shelves are overflowing with the latest dietary advice for an increasingly health-conscious public. Why, then, another book on diet and blood cholesterol?

That was certainly the question in my mind when Dr. Berns asked if I would review his manuscript. I was skeptical at first, but as I perused it, I quickly came to appreciate this book's great value and uniqueness. I also realized that sometimes it takes someone who, like Dr. Berns, has actually struggled with a cholesterol problem to ensure that sound nutritional advice is communicated in a practical and usable way.

The current explosion of information about what to eat to control your cholesterol level can confuse more than enlighten. That is precisely the reason this book is so important. Up to now authorities have asked you to do all these things: reduce cholesterol intake to less than 300 mg. per day or even 200 mg. per day, reduce total fat intake to less than 30 percent of calories, increase your carbohydrates to 50 to 60 percent of calories, reduce saturated fat to less than 10 percent of total calories, and so on. It's all sound information, but who can follow it all?

Buried deep in all that mixed advice, nevertheless, is the simple information that is the key to any cholesterol-lowering diet: (a) Saturated fat and cholesterol are the two components of the diet that raise the blood cholesterol level, (b) lowering your saturated fat and cholesterol consumption will act to lower your blood cholesterol level, and (c) of the two, saturated fat is the worse culprit. This cuts through all the controversial information and claims that have been confusing the public, and it is the simple and direct focus of this book.

Now, how do you, the average layperson, put this information to practical use? While there are already books that show the cholesterol and saturated fat content of foods, how can you judge the overall impact of each? Some foods are high in saturated fat but have little or no cholesterol (such as coconut), while others are high in cholesterol but have little saturated fat (such as shrimp). How can you compare different foods with their different combinations of saturated fat and cholesterol?

The answer lies in something called the *Cholesterol-Saturated Fat Index*, or *CSI*. The CSI for any given food is a number that takes into account both its saturated fat and its cholesterol content. The higher a food's CSI, the more it will raise the blood cholesterol level. Replacing high-CSI foods in your diet with low-CSI foods will reduce your cholesterol level. It has become that simple.

To my knowledge, this book represents the most exhaustive and comprehensive listing available of the CSI of foods. The book explains how to calculate the CSI yourself from information on product labels, labels that will be increasingly required in the 1990s.

Who can benefit from adopting a low-CSI diet? Certainly people with established coronary heart disease or people with elevated blood cholesterol or other risk factors (such as a family history of heart disease) that place them in jeopardy of developing a heart attack. If you already have an elevated blood cholesterol, dietary modification is the essential first step of therapy. In some instances a proper diet can spare individuals the need to take cholesterol-lowering drugs. But even if you require such medication, a proper diet is critical, as it permits the drugs to work most effectively and at the lowest possible doses.

Finally, there's good reason to recommend a lowered-CSI diet for almost anyone in the general population. In addition to its beneficial effects on blood cholesterol, a low-CSI, low-fat diet helps you reduce overweight, maintain ideal weight, and it may even reduce the risk of certain cancers.

In sum, a low-CSI diet is simply a healthier diet from which anyone can benefit. This book will show you how to achieve it.

ROBERT A. GELFAND, M.D., F.A.C.P.

Associate Clinical Professor of Medicine
Yale University School of Medicine

Director, Experimental Medicine
Department of Clinical Research
Pfizer Central Research

ROBERT A GELFAND, M.D., F.A.C.P. is a diplomat of the American Board of Internal Medicine and is certified in the subspecialty of endocrinology and metabolism. In his position at Pfizer Inc. he designs and directs the early clinical research programs involving new drug candidates for the treatment of lipid disorders. Dr. Gelfand also treats patients with lipid disorders at Yale University.

Introduction

THE PURPOSE OF THIS BOOK

This book introduces you to a new and far simpler way of choosing foods to bring down an elevated blood cholesterol level and maintain it at a heart-healthy level. Factors over which we have no control (heredity, for example) may predispose us to heart disease. That makes it very important to alter those factors we *can* control: adequate exercise, no smoking, treating high blood pressure, and a low-fat, low-cholesterol diet.

RELATIONSHIP OF CHOLESTEROL AND HEART DISEASE

A *low blood cholesterol level* is of critical importance in preventing heart attacks in both men and women. While there are multiple causes for a high cholesterol level, what you eat has a major effect upon it. One factor in preventing heart attacks that is under your control is to eat properly.

Your diet can raise your cholesterol level in two ways:

(A) By supplying too many calories

The most concentrated source of calories is fat, and Americans eat too much of it. We currently get 40 percent of our calories from fat, in significant contrast to health authorities' recommendation of under 30 percent. Some authorities even counsel a reduction to 20 percent.

(B) By eating foods high in *saturated fat* and *cholesterol*

These fats or fatty substances are the two principal food elements that you must avoid because they raise your blood cholesterol level.

Saturated fat is found in animal products (beef, fowl, fish, etc.) and in some nonanimal foods (some vegetable oils, nuts, seeds).

Cholesterol, a fatlike substance, exists only in animal products.

Eating foods with too much of either can lead to a deposit, called *plaque*, that builds up on the inside walls of the arteries. This is most serious when it begins to choke off the *coronary arteries* that supply blood to the heart. If a large enough coronary artery becomes blocked, a heart attack occurs. The higher the blood cholesterol above the recommended upper limit,* the more likely this will happen.

THE CHOLESTEROL-SATURATED FAT INDEX (CSI)

Some foods may contain either saturated fat or cholesterol, while many foods have both. High amounts of either, or both, can raise your blood cholesterol level. The confusion for most people comes when they try to judge foods that have both saturated fat and cholesterol in widely varying amounts.

For example, consider 4-ounce portions of three popular items in the American diet:

	grams of *saturated fat*	milligrams of *cholesterol*
steamed shrimp	0	221
London broil	3	110
prime roast beef (ribs 6-9)†	9	92

Which of these foods is most likely to raise your blood cholesterol level? Which is least likely to raise it?

The answer comes to us from *Lancet*, a leading medical journal, which in 1986 published a report about

---

*The ideal level for blood cholesterol is less than 200 mg. (milligrams, or thousandths of a gram) per dl. (deciliter, or tenth of a liter). When your doctor says your cholesterol level is 200, he or she is stating it in this standard form. The levels 200–240 are considered "borderline high." Over 240 is "definitely high."
†See page 150 Notes section on beef explaining "ribs 6–9."

research done at the medical school of the Oregon Health Sciences University in Portland. This article introduced a mathematical formula* combining both the saturated fat and cholesterol of a food into a *single index number*. This index number accurately reflects the ability of a food to raise the blood cholesterol level. It is called the

Cholesterol-Saturated Fat Index, or CSI.

This index makes choosing healthy foods quite simple: *The higher the CSI number, the more you should limit or avoid that food.***

Using the formula, here is the CSI for 4 oz. of each of the three foods we considered earlier:

	CSI
steamed shrimp	11
London broil, choice cut	7
roast beef, prime cut (ribs 6-9)†	14

You now know that the London broil is less likely to raise your cholesterol level than equal amounts of either the steamed shrimp or the roast ribs of beef. And you also know you'd be better off with an occasional 4 ounces of steamed shrimp than with the roast beef.

*The actual formula appears on page 171 in the Appendix.
**Fish are the one exception. See later in the "Notes" section, page 152.
†See page 150 Notes section on beef explaining "ribs 6–9."

THE AMOUNT OF ANY FOOD YOU EAT AND THE CSI

The amount of any food consumed can make a big difference. Let's compare two foods with quite different CSI numbers:

4 oz. of roast chicken, light meat (no skin), CSI = 6

versus

1 cup (5 oz.) of vanilla ice cream, CSI = 15

If you were to eat three times the 4-ounce portion of chicken, for a total of 12 ounces, the CSI number would change to

3 times the CSI of 6 = CSI of 18

Conclusion: Eating that large a portion of white meat chicken, 12 ounces, CSI = 18, risks elevating your cholesterol level more than one cup of ice cream, CSI = 15.

There is no such thing as a "good" food or a "bad" food. Rather, it all depends on the *CSI*, the *number of calories*, and the *total fat*. And all three of these numbers, in turn, may change depending on the *amount* of any food you eat.

Incidentally, watch out for restaurant portions. Servings of meat can be quite large, commonly ranging between 8 to 16 ounces.

TOTALING THE CSI NUMBERS FOR A MEAL

To get the total CSI for a meal, just add up the CSI numbers for each food in the meal, taking portion size into account. To learn your total CSI for the day, add together the CSIs for each meal and any other snacks and beverages you consume that day.

Breakfast example:*

	CSI Number
6 oz. orange juice	0
2 large poached chicken eggs	24
2 slices of toast	0
1 tablsp. butter on toast	9
1 cup of coffee	0
½ oz. light cream in the coffee	3
TOTAL BREAKFAST CSI	36

Lunch example:

cheeseburger (4 oz. meat, 1 oz. cheese)	19
fast-food French fries (10 strips)	3
milk shake (16 fl. oz.)	8
TOTAL LUNCH CSI	30

Dinner example:

roast prime ribs of beef (6 oz.)	21
mashed potatoes (½ cup)	0
made with milk and butter	2

*For explanations of measurements and conversion tables, see "Common Measures" on pp. 14–15.

string beans	0
with 1 tsp. butter	3
salad	0
with 1 tblsp. oil and vinegar	2
chocolate cake, fudge frosting (3 oz.)	6
1 cup of coffee	0
with ½ oz. light cream	2
TOTAL DINNER CSI	36
TOTAL CSI FOR THE DAY	102

CSI GOALS

Each meal above has a very high CSI, higher than many people should have as a total for the entire day! But don't despair—you will find in the table of foods beginning on page 19 that there are a great many very good, very low CSI foods to eat. In addition, there are all the fruits, vegetables, grains, pastas, and other starches we don't include in the table of foods because, with a very few exceptions (see footnote 3 on page 17), they have a CSI of *zero*!

Starting on page 164, we show you how to choose a CSI goal based on your caloric intake and the degree of fat restriction you want to achieve. Don't be put off by all the numbers you see there. You'll find these tables very simple to use.

DEALING WITH CHANGING YOUR DIET

First, is it really all worthwhile? Well, consider the following:

> A recent study shows that *even late in life*, and *even after a heart attack*, a diet low in saturated fat and cholesterol can diminish fatty deposits choking coronary arteries.

> The National Academy of Sciences recently reviewed nearly *ten thousand* research papers on the relationship of diet to heart disease. Their conclusion: A diet high in saturated fat and cholesterol is of major importance in causing heart disease.

Don't be misled by the occasional sensational newspaper story, usually quoting some preliminary report, saying that all the medical and dietetic authorities are wrong or that the effect of diet on the cholesterol level or the effect of the cholesterol level on heart attacks has really not been demonstrated. For the vast majority of scientists, the National Academy of Sciences review has put the matter to rest: Diet does count, and a high blood cholesterol level is a serious risk to health.

A GRADUAL COURSE OF ACTION

Once you've set your first CSI goal, don't feel you must achieve it right away. In fact, you'll be far better off working *gradually* toward that goal. Experience shows that adapting by degrees to new tastes makes for greater acceptance of them. Take it in steps: If you use whole milk (3.3 percent fat), don't switch directly to skim milk; rather, try several weeks of 2 percent milk, a few weeks of 1 percent milk, and then skim milk.

Should you weaken and splurge one day, you're *not* a failure. Don't give up! Just make it up by finding foods with low CSI numbers for your next meals. That way you can still achieve a low CSI total for that period.

If doing it all at once—setting a CSI target, totaling the calories, and calculating the total fat—seems overwhelming, take the easiest step first, a gradual shifting toward foods with lower CSIs. You'll get an immediate benefit since the lower you go with your total daily CSI, the lower your intake will be of saturated fat, total fat, cholesterol, and calories. Remember that each and every step you take down the CSI scale means less risk to your heart.

TOTAL CALORIES AND TOTAL FAT

When you get close to your CSI target, even though it's probable you'll be eating properly, do check out the *calories* and *total fat* to be sure. We show you how to do this in the Appendix, starting on page 151. Keep in mind that even though some foods have a relatively low CSI, they may still supply a large number of calories and fat. Peanuts and peanut butter are examples of this. They have a relatively low CSI (2 CSI for a 1-ounce portion) but contain a considerable amount of nonsaturated fats and are thus high-fat, high-calorie foods. No matter how low your CSI, a high-fat diet or just being overweight can still cause an elevated blood cholesterol level.

You may have heard about HDL, often referred to as the "good" cholesterol, and LDL, often called the "bad" cholesterol. These are actually cholesterol-carrying particles in the blood stream.

Researchers believe HDL can remove plaque that has built up inside arteries and take it back to the liver to be disposed of. When this happens in the coronary arteries, it reduces the risk of a heart attack. In contrast, LDL seems to carry cholesterol from the liver to the arteries to form more plaque, thereby increasing the risk of a heart attack.

The more saturated fat and cholesterol you eat, the more likely you will create a dangerous combination of low HDL and high LDL. In addition to limiting saturated fat and cholesterol in your diet, you may raise HDL and lower LDL if you lose excess weight, exercise, and stop smoking. A modest daily amount of alcohol (say, one glass of wine with dinner) may also raise the HDL.

If your total blood cholesterol count is high, your doctor will probably request a blood test to measure both HDL and LDL.

Following a heart-healthy diet is simple now because of the CSI, the Cholesterol-Saturated Fat Index. Changing to a low-CSI diet costs nothing, and you'll still eat well while reducing your chances of a heart attack. If you are overweight, you'll probably lose weight, feel better, and look better too. Best of all, the payoff starts the day you begin!

How to Use This Book

THE TABLE OF FOODS

The Table of Foods lists generic foods and, very occasionally, brand-name foods. Foods are listed alphabetically.

On the *left* side of the table is a column labeled *CSI 4 oz.* This column presents the CSI for a standard 4-ounce weight for every food. It allows you to directly compare the CSI for each food in *equal amounts* by weight. By referring to the standard 4-ounce CSI column, you can see the basic ability of each food to raise your blood cholesterol level.

To the *right* of the food names we show the *CSI, TOTAL CALORIES*, and *TOTAL FAT* content of *common portions* of each food. Common portions are often more or less than 4 ounces, and may be measured by *weight or volume*. (Weight is in ounces only. Volume measures may be cups, tablespoons, fluid ounces, etc.)

ADJUSTING FOR YOUR "USUAL PORTION"

What if the portion you usually eat, your "*usual portion*," differs from the *common portion* shown? Simply weigh your *usual portion* on a mail or food scale and calculate the difference. We show you how to do this in the Appendix on page 168.

FOUR STEPS TO TAKE

1. Find your *Desirable Weight* on page 162 of the Appendix.

2. Select your *Recommended Average Caloric Intake* on pages 164–165 of the Appendix.

3. Choose your daily CSI goal on page 167 of the Appendix. (You may find it convenient to make individual CSI targets for breakfast, lunch, and dinner.)

4. Select foods from the Table of Foods beginning on page 19, keeping in mind that most fruits, vegetables, grains and flour products, and rice dishes have a CSI of 0, however large their portion, provided that they are not prepared with fats, eggs, or other items with a higher CSI count.

Common Measures

VOLUME MEASURES

3 tsp. = 1 tblsp.
1 tblsp. = ½ fluid ounce (fl. oz.)
8 tblsp. = ½ cup

1 cup = 8 fluid ounces (fl. oz.)
1 pint = 2 cups
1 quart = 2 pints

> N.B.: *fluid ounces* (fl. oz.) are a *volume* measure, not to be confused with *oz.* (ounces), which is the *weight* of something measured on a scale. The weight of a *fluid ounce* depends on its density. For example, a fluid ounce of tomato soup would weigh a lot more on a scale than would a fluid ounce of plain water.

WEIGHT MEASURES

1 cup of water = 8 ounces (oz.)
1 oz. = 28.4 grams (gms.)
4 oz. = 113.4 grams

1 pound (lb.) = 16 ounces = 454 grams
1 gram = .035 ounce

Abbreviations

" = inches (example: 3" = three inches)
oz. = ounce(s)
gms. = grams
fl. oz. = fluid ounce(s)
qt. = quart
tsp. = teaspoon
tblsp. = tablespoon

USDA = United States Department of Agriculture

? = data not available

NOTE: we rounded off all numbers to whole numbers to make the tables easier to read. This makes for insignificant differences in table values.

Footnotes to The Table

(1) Method of cooking unspecified.

(2) *¼ pie* refers to a slice equal to one-quarter of a pizza pie 14 inches in diameter.

(3) Some groups of foods are not listed because almost all in that group would have a CSI number of 0. We thus omit

fruits (except avocado)
flour (including plain pastas and simple breads)
grains
rice
vegetables

But we do list foods from these groups if common preparations involve oils, eggs, coconut, etc., that cause the CSI to climb. For example, potatoes have a CSI = 0, but frying them in oil or lard causes a significant CSI increase; some breads contain eggs; etc. Obviously, the more CSI = 0 foods you can include in your diet, the healthier your diet will be.

See the remarks about *pasta* on page 154 in the Notes section.

(4) Light mayonnaise figures are a mean average for three common commercial light mayonnaise preparations. Check the labels when purchasing light mayonnaise for the lowest combination of total fat, saturated fat, and calories.

(5) Dessert pie figures are for one-eighth of a 9-inch-diameter pie.

THE TABLE OF FOODS

-A-

	abalone (see shellfish)
	Alexander, brandy (see cocktail)
	aspic (see salad)
3	almond paste...
5	anchovies, smoked ....
	animal crackers (see crackers)
	avocado (see vegetable)

-B-

	bacon
6	Canadian, grilled...
25	cured, roasted, broiled, or pan-fried.............
	bagel
3	egg ....
0	plain or flavored ....
12	baklava...
4	barley, pilaf...
	beans, baked or refried (see vegetable, beans)
	*beef
117	brains, pan-fried...
120	simmered ....

*See entry in Notes section for this class of food.

COMMON PORTION

AMOUNT	CSI	TOTAL CALORIES	TOTAL FAT GRAMS
1 oz.	**1**	127	8
6 fillets	**1**	50	2
2 oz.	**3**	105	5
3 slices	**4**	109	9
1	**2**	225	4
1	**0**	225	2
2 oz.	**6**	312	21
1 cup	**8**	290	13
4 oz.	**117**	222	18
4 oz.	**120**	181	14

*beef (cont.)
     brisket
8   flat half, braised...
11   point half, braised...
     calf items (see calf)
7   chipped ....
9   chuck, arm pot roast, all grades, braised.....
12   blade roast, all grades, braised ....
13   corned (cured)...
     corned beef hash (see hash)
     filet (see beef, tenderloin)
10   flank, braised or broiled...............................
13   ground, lean, baked, broiled, or pan-fried ...
12   extra lean, baked, broiled, or pan-fried (see
            also hamburger) ....
13   heart, simmered...
8   jerky..
23   kidneys, simmered ....
24   liver, braised...
31   pan-fried ....
     loin (see short loin and top loin)
     London broil (see beef, round, top round)
17   lungs, braised ....
     macaroni and beef casserole (see casserole)

*See entry in Notes section for this class of food.

COMMON PORTION

AMOUNT	CSI	TOTAL CALORIES	TOTAL FAT GRAMS
4 oz.	8	246	11
4 oz.	11	277	16
4 oz.	7	231	7
4 oz.	9	237	9
4 oz.	12	286	15
4 oz.	13	283	21
4 oz.	10	267	15
4 oz.	13	307	21
4 oz.	12	286	18
4 oz.	13	197	6
2 oz.	4	106	6
4 oz.	23	162	4
4 oz.	24	182	6
4 oz.	31	245	9
4 oz.	17	136	4

	*beef (cont.)
	meatballs and meat loaf (see under these names)
15	oxtails ....
	porterhouse steak (see short loin)
	pot roast (see beef, round, bottom round)
	prime ribs (see beef, ribs 6-12)
	rib, eye, small end (ribs 10-12)
9	select, broiled or roasted...........................
10	choice, broiled or roasted..........................
12	prime, broiled or roasted...........................
9	rib, whole, (ribs 6-12)
	select, broiled or roasted...........................
11	choice, broiled or roasted..........................
14	prime, broiled or roasted...........................
10	rib, large end, (ribs 6-9)
	select, broiled or roasted...........................
11	choice, broiled or roasted..........................
14	prime, broiled or roasted...........................
	ribs, short (see beef, short ribs)
9	round: bottom round, choice, braised...........
7	choice, roasted..
8	pot roast, braised ....
6	eye of round, all grades, broiled or roasted..

*See entry in Notes section for this class of food.

COMMON PORTION

AMOUNT	CSI	TOTAL CALORIES	TOTAL FAT GRAMS
4 oz.	**15**	328	21
4 oz.	**9**	223	10
4 oz.	**10**	254	13
4 oz.	**12**	294	18
4 oz.	**9**	233	12
4 oz.	**11**	267	16
4 oz.	**14**	317	21
4 oz.	**10**	249	13
4 oz.	**11**	286	17
4 oz.	**14**	321	21
4 oz.	**9**	241	10
4 oz.	**7**	207	8
4 oz.	**8**	218	9
4 oz.	**6**	188	5

*beef (cont.)

8	full cut, broiled or roasted......................
7	tip round, choice or select, roasted..........
9	prime, broiled or roasted......................
	top round
7	choice, braised or broiled........................
7	select, braised or broiled........................
8	choice, pan-fried ....
8	prime, broiled or roasted........................
	salami (see salami, beef)
7	shank, crosscuts, simmered......................
	short loin
9	porterhouse steak, choice, broiled ....
14	T-bone steak, choice, broiled....................
	top loin
9	choice, broiled.................................
11	prime, broiled.................................
7	select, broiled.................................
14	short ribs, braised ....
8	sirloin, top, select, roasted........................
	stew (see stew)
13	Stroganoff, typical..................................
	tenderloin
9	select or choice, broiled...........................

*See entry in Notes section for this class of food.

COMMON PORTION

AMOUNT	CSI	TOTAL CALORIES	TOTAL FAT GRAMS
4 oz.	8	311	21
4 oz.	7	203	7
4 oz.	9	241	11
4 oz.	7	223	7
4 oz.	7	203	4
4 oz.	8	257	10
4 oz.	8	243	10
4 oz.	7	227	7
4 oz.	9	246	12
4 oz.	14	336	24
4 oz.	9	235	11
4 oz.	11	277	15
4 oz.	7	209	8
4 oz.	14	334	20
4 oz.	8	204	6
1 cup	27	571	44
4 oz.	9	243	12

	*beef (cont.)
10	prime, broiled...
16	tongue, simmered...
8	top loin, broiled...
8	top sirloin, all grades, broiled......................
	tournedos (see beef, tenderloin)
	T-bone steak (see beef, short loin)
7	tripe...
	vegetable stew (see stew, beef vegetable)
6	**beefalo**, composite of cuts, roasted..................
	beer salami or beerwurst (see salami)
14	**biscuit**, plain (from buttermilk dough)............
6	**bison**, roasted...
	blintz (see crepe)
22	**blood pudding**...
	bologna
17	beef ....
11	pork..
10	turkey...
	brains (see beef, calf, pork)
5	**bran**, rice (crude) ....
14	**bratwurst**, pork, cooked................................
22	**braunschweiger**..

*See entry in Notes section for this class of food.

COMMON PORTION

AMOUNT	CSI	TOTAL CALORIES	TOTAL FAT GRAMS
4 oz.	10	233	11
4 oz.	16	322	24
4 oz.	8	321	23
4 oz.	8	215	8
4 oz.	7	113	5
4 oz.	6	213	7
2 oz.	7	213	10
4 oz.	6	162	3
3 oz.	16	324	29
2 oz.	9	177	16
2 oz.	6	141	11
2 oz.	5	122	9
2 oz.	2	180	12
2 oz.	7	170	14
2 oz.	11	204	18

bread (see footnote 3, page 17)
(see also under names like "brioche" and "popover")

4	Boboli ....
7	challah..
8	cheese ....
10	corn bread (typical) ....
7	egg ....
2	focaccia...
4	nut ....
10	pumpkin, no nuts ....
	pudding (see pudding)
1	white, firm..
8	zucchini, no nuts..
15	**brioche** ....
	broccoli quiche (see vegetable, broccoli)
15	**brotwurst**, pork & beef...................................
	brownies
7	(shortening 19%, dry milk 6%)....................
13	frosted, typical ....
1	unfrosted, from mix, oil, no nuts, egg white.
7	from scratch (shortening, egg whites, chocolate, nuts) ....
14	typical (shortening, chocolate, nuts, whole eggs) ....

COMMON PORTION

AMOUNT	CSI	TOTAL CALORIES	TOTAL FAT GRAMS
2 oz.	1	173	8
2 oz.	5	207	5
2 oz.	4	174	6
2 oz.	5	190	8
2 oz.	4	207	5
2 oz.	1	180	5
2 oz.	2	199	10
2 oz.	5	203	6
2 oz.	0	151	2
2 oz.	4	229	12
1 oz.	4	119	6
4 oz.	15	366	32
4 oz.	7	458	19
4 oz.	13	484	28
4 oz.	1	439	12
4 oz.	7	475	27
4 oz.	14	497	30

burrito
8   beef ....
4   beans ....
71   **butter** ....
6   almond ....
11   cashew ....
72   whipped ....
       peanut (see peanut butter)
       sesame (see tahini)
buttermilk (see milk, buttermilk)
butterscotch (see under candy or chips)

-C-

cabbage roll
4   ground beef, rice..
4   with rice and cheese..
café au lait (see coffee)
cake
0   angel food (unfrosted, unglazed)...................
8   carrot (unfrosted, unglazed) ....
23   cheesecake, typical (unfrosted, unglazed)....
10   chiffon (unfrosted, unglazed).......................
           chocolate
8   chocolate fudge frosting...........................

32

COMMON PORTION

AMOUNT	CSI	TOTAL CALORIES	TOTAL FAT GRAMS
4 oz.	8	320	15
4 oz.	4	233	7
1 tblsp.	9	101	11
1 tblsp.	1	101	9
1 tblsp.	2	94	8
1 tblsp.	9	81	9
4 oz.	4	144	7
3 oz.	3	120	8
3 oz.	0	201	0
3 oz.	6	286	13
3 oz.	17	275	19
3 oz.	7	273	11
3 oz.	6	256	9

cake (cont.)

10	chocolate pudding (unfrosted, unglazed)..
6	"7-minute" frosting......................................

devil's food

11	7-minute frosting......................................
12	typical, chocolate fudge frosting...............
9	fruitcake (unfrosted, unglazed) ....
7	gingerbread (unfrosted, unglazed).................
6	jelly roll, all flavors except chocolate (unfrosted, unglazed) ....
18	chocolate, cream filling (unfrosted, unglazed) ....

pound

19	typical (unfrosted, unglazed)......................
19	chocolate, typical (unfrosted, unglazed)...
8	shortcake...
5	spice, typical (unfrosted, unglazed)..............
14	sponge (unfrosted, unglazed) ....
12	trifle (pound cake, fruit, jam, custard).........

white

3	egg whites, cocoa frosting ....
5	egg whites, chocolate fudge frosting........
8	homemade (milk and butter), chocolate fudge frosting...................................

COMMON PORTION

AMOUNT	CSI	TOTAL CALORIES	TOTAL FAT GRAMS
3 oz.	7	351	14
3 oz.	4	231	6
3 oz.	8	301	12
3 oz.	9	316	13
3 oz.	7	296	12
3 oz.	5	208	6
3 oz.	5	238	1
3 oz.	14	292	11
3 oz.	14	361	18
3 oz.	14	402	21
3 oz.	6	184	9
3 oz.	4	240	9
3 oz.	10	243	3
3 oz.	9	190	13
3 oz.	2	226	6
3 oz.	3	227	7
3 oz.	6	272	10

4	pudding (unfrosted, unglazed).....................
10	yellow pudding (unfrosted, unglazed)..........
8	zucchini, typical (unfrosted, unglazed).........

calf

147	brains (preparation not specified).................
52	kidney (preparation not specified)................
21	liver (preparation not specified)...................

canneloni (see footnote 3, page 17)

canola oil (see oil)

*****candy**

18	almond roca..
4	butterscotch..
12	caramel, plain and chocolate ....
12	cherries, chocolate-covered ....
21	chocolate, milk type ....
12	creams, chocolate-covered.............................
6	fudge...
6	with walnuts..
16	malted milk balls ....
4	nut brittle..
4	peanuts, carob-coated......................................
6	pecan praline ....
	raisins
3	carob-coated ....
12	chocolate-covered..

*See entry in Notes section for this class of food.

COMMON PORTION

AMOUNT	CSI	TOTAL CALORIES	TOTAL FAT GRAMS
3 oz.	3	230	9
3 oz.	7	351	14
3 oz.	6	285	9
4 oz.	147	156	11
4 oz.	52	286	13
4 oz.	21	204	5
2 oz.	9	305	21
2 oz.	2	226	18
2 oz.	6	232	10
2 oz.	6	246	10
2 oz.	6	240	10
2 oz.	6	246	10
2 oz.	3	230	6
2 oz.	3	257	10
2 oz.	8	270	14
2 oz.	2	302	15
2 oz.	2	280	16
2 oz.	3	243	9
2 oz.	2	224	8
2 oz.	6	240	10

	*candy (cont.)
8	toffee......................................
	(candies without additives that raise the CSI are omitted)
	cappuccino (see coffee)
	caramel (see candy)
8	caribou, roasted.............................
0	carob, powder mix for milk..............
	casserole
4	beef and macaroni (goulash type)..............
5	chicken rice...................................
6	hamburger rice ....
2	tuna noodle, typical ....
6	zucchini...
39	caviar ....
	cereal
1	granola, low-fat, commercial ....
17	with coconut oil, commercial ....
3	with soy oil, commercial ....
	Chateaubriand (see beef, tenderloin)
	cheese
28	American, processed........................
26	bleu (blue)...................................
24	brie...
22	Camembert ....

*See entry in Notes section for this class of food.

COMMON PORTION

AMOUNT	CSI	TOTAL CALORIES	TOTAL FAT GRAMS
2 oz.	4	226	6
4 oz.	8	189	5
1 oz.	0	107	0
1 cup	9	328	9
1 cup	10	311	16
1 cup	12	385	24
1 cup	5	321	15
4 oz.	6	72	5
1 tblsp.	6	81	6
1 cup	1	250	6
1 cup	17	503	20
1 cup	3	495	18
1 oz.	7	106	9
1 oz.	6	100	8
1 oz.	6	95	8
1 oz.	5	85	7

CSI 4 oz.	
	cheese (cont.)
30	cheddar ....
	cottage
1	dry curd ....
1	1% "low-fat" ....
2	2% "low-fat" ....
4	4% ....
	cream
15	light...
32	regular...
30	whipped ....
	(see also Neufchatel below)
32	Edam..
22	feta ....
27	Gouda ....
28	Gruyère ....
32	Limburger ....
	mozzarella
20	regular...
4	imitation (made with vegetable oil instead of butterfat) ....
16	part skim ....
28	Muenster ....
32	Monterey jack ....
22	Neufchatel..

COMMON PORTION

AMOUNT	CSI	TOTAL CALORIES	TOTAL FAT GRAMS
1 oz.	8	114	9
4 oz.	1	97	1
4 oz.	1	81	1
4 oz.	2	102	2
4 oz.	4	120	5
1 oz.	4	60	5
1 oz.	8	99	10
1 oz.	8	100	10
1 oz.	8	114	9
1 oz.	6	75	6
1 oz.	7	101	8
1 oz.	6	107	8
1 oz.	8	114	9
1 oz.	5	80	6
1 oz.	1	80	6
1 oz.	4	72	5
1 oz.	7	104	9
1 oz.	8	114	9
1 oz.	5	74	7

cheese (cont.)
   Parmesan
23   hard..
27   grated..
32   Port du Salut...
24   provolone...
   ricotta
7   part skim ....
12   whole milk ....
32   Roquefort...
19   spread, American cheese type.....................
   Swiss
26   regular..
15   processed ....
10 **cheese puffs**...
cheesecake (see cake)
*****chicken**, broiler
   back meat
8   stewed..
9   roasted..
10   pan-fried ....
   breast (see under light meat)
11   breast and wing, breaded and pan-fried.......
   dark meat
7   stewed..

COMMON PORTION

AMOUNT	CSI	TOTAL CALORIES	TOTAL FAT GRAMS
1 oz.	6	131	7
1 tblsp.	1	23	2
1 oz.	8	100	8
1 oz.	6	100	8
1 oz.	2	39	2
1 oz.	3	49	4
1 oz.	8	114	9
1 oz.	5	83	6
1 oz.	6	107	8
1 oz.	4	95	7
2 cups	3	190	12
4 oz.	8	237	13
4 oz.	9	271	15
4 oz.	10	327	17
4 oz.	11	344	21
4 oz.	7	204	9

	*chicken (cont.)
8	roasted...
9	pan-fried ....
	drumstick
7	roasted or stewed...............................
8	pan-fried ....
12	drumstick and thigh, breaded and fried.......
24	giblets, simmered...............................
12	gizzard, simmered...............................
16	heart, simmered.................................
	light meat
6	roasted...
6	stewed...
7	pan-fried ....
38	liver, simmered..................................
7	neck, simmered ....
	thigh
8	stewed...
9	pan-fried ....
9	roasted...
	wing
6	stewed...
7	roasted...
8	pan-fried ....
4	cacciatore, typical ....

*See entry in Notes section for this class of food.

COMMON PORTION

AMOUNT	CSI	TOTAL CALORIES	TOTAL FAT GRAMS
4 oz.	8	232	11
4 oz.	9	271	13
4 oz.	7	194	6
4 oz.	8	221	9
4 oz.	12	330	20
2 oz.	12	89	3
2 oz.	6	87	2
2 oz.	8	105	4
4 oz.	6	196	5
4 oz.	6	180	5
4 oz.	7	218	6
2 oz.	19	89	3
4 oz.	7	203	9
4 oz.	8	221	11
4 oz.	9	247	12
4 oz.	9	237	12
4 oz.	6	205	8
4 oz.	7	230	9
4 oz.	8	239	10
4 oz.	4	152	8

*chicken (cont.)

27	capon, giblets, simmered................................
9	Parmesan..

roaster

7	dark meat..
6	light meat ....
22	giblets, simmered ....
5	roll, light meat ....
10	stewer, dark meat, stewed............................

chile relleno (see relleno)

chili

1	chicken, with beans ....
5	con carne, with beans, canned.....................

chips

29	butterscotch...
3	carob ....
18	chocolate..
6	corn ....
10	potato ....
9	taro..

tortilla

10	fried in lard..
20	fried in palm or coconut oil ....
4	fried in corn oil ....
20	**chitterlings**, simmered ....

*See entry in Notes section for this class of food.

COMMON PORTION

AMOUNT	CSI	TOTAL CALORIES	TOTAL FAT GRAMS
2 oz.	13	93	3
4 oz.	9	310	24
4 oz.	7	202	10
4 oz.	6	174	5
2 oz.	11	94	3
4 oz.	5	180	8
4 oz.	10	293	17
1 cup	1	190	4
1 cup	5	282	14
1 oz.	7	151	9
1 oz.	1	116	2
1 oz.	5	129	6
2 cups	4	370	22
10 chips	2	105	7
1 cup	2	114	6
2 cups	5	282	12
2 cups	10	282	12
2 cups	2	282	12
4 oz.	20	344	32

chocolate
  baking
24   sweetened (German) ....
24   semisweet ....
36   unsweetened ....
  hot milk drink (see milk, cocoa)
chocolate candy (see candy)
chocolate chips (see chips)
3 **chocolate malt** powder mix for milk ....
chocolate milk (see milk, chocolate)
chocolate sauce (see sauce, chocolate)
chocolate syrup (see syrup, chocolate)
chowder (see soup, clam chowder, etc.)
chow mein
7   chicken...
12   pork...
clams (see shellfish)
2 **cobbler**, fruit, biscuit topping..........................
cocoa (see milk, cocoa)
cocktail
6   Alexander, brandy ....
5   crème de menthe...
5   grasshopper..
8   piña colada ....
4 **cocoa**, dry powder...

COMMON PORTION

AMOUNT	CSI	TOTAL CALORIES	TOTAL FAT GRAMS
1 oz.	6	148	10
1 oz.	6	144	10
1 oz.	9	143	15
1 oz.	1	107	1
1 cup	4	224	9
1 cup	7	270	15
1 cup	2	272	8
6 oz.	9	417	12
6 oz.	9	537	12
6 oz.	9	537	12
6 oz.	13	323	14
1 tblsp.	1	14	1

	cocoa drink (see milk, cocoa)
	coconut (see nuts, coconut)
1	**coffee**, café au lait or cappuccino or mocha or Vienna..
7	**coffee cake**, streusel topping ....
	coleslaw
4	salad dressing...
6	mayonnaise...
	conch (see shellfish, conch)
	cookies
4	arrowroot baby..
12	chocolate chip
	commercial, giant size...............................
11	typical homemade......................................
13	typical commercial.....................................
12	commercial, typical deli ....
7	fig bars, commercial....................................
5	fortune...
5	gingersnaps, commercial ....
11	oatmeal, commercial....................................
4	typical homemade ....
13	Oreos, commercial.......................................
12	peanut butter, typical homemade....................
11	pecan shortbread, commercial.........................
14	sugar, typical homemade...............................

COMMON PORTION

AMOUNT	CSI	TOTAL CALORIES	TOTAL FAT GRAMS
1 cup	3	85	3
3"×3"×2"	6	316	12
1 cup	4	201	19
1 cup	6	282	29
2 oz.	2	227	9
4 oz.	12	564	28
2 oz.	8	240	16
2 oz.	6	282	13
2 oz.	6	283	13
2 oz.	4	238	5
1 cookie	0	34	1
2 oz.	3	238	5
2 oz.	6	282	14
2 oz.	3	285	14
2 oz.	6	282	13
2 oz.	6	254	14
2 oz.	5	269	5
2 oz.	7	230	10

8	vanilla wafers, commercial ....
15	**coquille Saint Jacques** (containing 3 oz. cooked scallops) ....
	corn dog (see frankfurter)
	corn oil (see oil)
	corn bread (see bread)
	corned beef (see beef, corned)
	Cornish game hen
8	dark meat (see footnote 1, page 17)............
5	white meat (see footnote 1, page 17)..........
	cottage cheese (see cheese, cottage)
	crab
3	Alaska king, steamed.....................................
10	baked (in flour, egg 2%)................................
10	blue, cake (egg 9%, margarine for frying 5%) ....
5	canned...
6	steamed ....
3	Dungeness, raw ....
3	queen, raw ....
6	soft-shell, pan-fried.......................................
	crackers
5	animal ....
2	graham ....
6	soda, most brands ....

COMMON PORTION

AMOUNT	CSI	TOTAL CALORIES	TOTAL FAT GRAMS
2 oz.	1	238	5
9 oz.	34	528	41
4 oz.	8	222	9
4 oz.	5	186	4
4 oz.	3	110	2
4 oz.	10	167	2
4 oz.	10	176	9
4 oz.	5	112	1
4 oz.	6	116	2
4 oz.	3	98	1
4 oz.	3	102	1
4 oz.	6	303	16
8 small	1	91	2
3 regular	0	83	2
six	1	79	2

CSI 4 oz.	
10	**crayfish**, mixed species, steamed......................
	cream
18	light...
22	medium (25% fat)..
35	heavy..
10	half-and-half ....
	imitation (see creamer)
	Irish (see liqueur)
11	sour, half-and-half, cultured ....
10	sour, light (10% fat).....................................
17	sour, regular (20% fat).................................
28	whipping...
	whipped
23	from aerosol can, dairy cream..................
19	from aerosol can, nondairy imitation ("topping")......................................
16	**cream puff**..
	creamer
	coffee, nondairy
2	soybean oil...
11	coconut oil...
39	powdered, nondairy ....
	crepe
12	blintz type ....
8	typical..

COMMON PORTION

AMOUNT	CSI	TOTAL CALORIES	TOTAL FAT GRAMS
4 oz.	**10**	129	2
1 tblsp.	**2**	29	3
1 tblsp.	**3**	37	4
1 tblsp.	**5**	52	6
1 tblsp.	**1**	18	2
2 tblsp.	**3**	40	4
2 tblsp.	**5**	90	6
2 tblsp.	**9**	117	12
2 tblsp.	**7**	83	9
2 tblsp.	**2**	21	2
2 tblsp.	**1**	20	2
3 oz.	**12**	173	8
1 tblsp.	**0**	19	1
1 tblsp.	**1**	19	1
1 tblsp.	**2**	33	2
4 oz.	**12**	227	14
4 oz.	**8**	193	7

19	**croissant**...
19	**croutons**, commercial....................................
9	**custard**, baked...

-D-

	Danish (see pastry)
	deer (see venison)
	dip
3	bean...
22	cheese ....
13	clam ....
19	shrimp...
17	sour cream.......................................
17	spinach..
	doughnut
5	unfrosted...
8	frosted...
11	frosted with coconut.......................
	dressing (see salad dressing)
10	**duck**, domestic or wild, roasted, eaten without skin ....

COMMON PORTION

AMOUNT	CSI	TOTAL CALORIES	TOTAL FAT GRAMS
one	9	167	12
½ cup	3	89	4
½ cup	11	150	7
¼ cup	2	82	3
¼ cup	8	118	10
¼ cup	6	87	7
¼ cup	8	99	8
¼ cup	8	111	11
¼ cup	4	138	13
1 3-inch	4	153	6
1 3-inch	5	279	10
1 3-inch	7	309	12
4 oz.	10	228	13

-E-

10	**eclair**, chocolate..
	eel (see fish)
	egg, chicken, large
32	deviled, typical..
23	omelet (margarine 4%), plain ....
31	pan-fried in margarine....................................
28	poached or boiled ....
24	scrambled (milk 22%), cooked in margarine.
0	white only ....
84	yolk only, raw..
26	**egg Benedict**..
54	**egg**, duck, boiled or poached ....
15	**egg foo young** ....
7	**egg roll** (with shrimp and pork)......................
52	**egg**, quail, boiled or poached ....
8	**eggnog** (no alcohol) ....
5	**elk**, roasted...
	enchilada
9	beef ....
12	cheese ....
7	chicken..
	English muffin (see muffin)

COMMON PORTION

AMOUNT	CSI	TOTAL CALORIES	TOTAL FAT GRAMS
4 oz.	10	201	10
1 egg	16	130	12
2 large	25	184	14
2 large	25	182	14
2 large	24	148	10
2 large	26	202	15
2 large	0	34	0
2 large	25	118	10
1	30	238	11
2 eggs	68	260	19
3 oz.	10	143	13
1 roll	6	158	11
2 eggs	8	28	2
1 cup	19	342	19
4 oz.	5	165	2
4 oz.	9	256	17
4 oz.	12	256	17
4 oz.	7	197	10

-F-

3	**falafel** ....
15	**fetuccini Alfredo**...
	filet mignon (see beef, tenderloin)
	*fish
	bass
5	freshwater, raw....................................
4	sea, mixed species, broiled ....
5	striped, broiled ....
4	bluefish, broiled ....
4	burbot, raw ....
6	carp, broiled ....
	catfish, channel
4	broiled...
8	breaded with egg, milk, and cornmeal, pan-fried..................................
4	cisco, smoked..
	cod
	Atlantic
3	broiled...
9	dried and salted....................................
3	Pacific, raw ....
	croaker, Atlantic
9	breaded with egg and milk and pan-fried.

*See entry in Notes section for this class of food.

COMMON PORTION

AMOUNT	CSI	TOTAL CALORIES	TOTAL FAT GRAMS
4 oz.	3	378	20
4 oz.	15	278	19
4 oz.	5	129	4
4 oz.	4	140	3
4 oz.	5	109	3
4 oz.	4	139	5
4 oz.	4	101	1
4 oz.	6	184	8
4 oz.	4	132	5
4 oz.	8	258	15
4 oz.	4	201	13
4 oz.	3	118	1
4 oz.	9	108	1
4 oz.	3	93	1
4 oz.	9	250	14

	*fish (cont.)
5	raw
4	dolphin, raw
5	drum, freshwater, raw
13	eel, broiled
	flatfish
4	broiled
5	filet, breaded with egg and milk, pan-fried
2	gefilte fish with broth
3	grouper, broiled
	haddock
4	broiled
5	smoked
	halibut
3	Atlantic and Pacific, broiled
5	Greenland, raw
	herring
	Atlantic
5	kippered
3	pickled
3	broiled
8	Pacific, raw
	mackerel
9	Atlantic, broiled

*See entry in Notes section for this class of food.

COMMON PORTION

AMOUNT	CSI	TOTAL CALORIES	TOTAL FAT GRAMS
4 oz.	5	118	4
4 oz.	4	97	1
4 oz.	5	134	6
4 oz.	13	266	17
4 oz.	4	132	2
4 oz.	5	263	14
4 oz.	2	35	1
4 oz.	3	133	1
4 oz.	4	126	1
4 oz.	5	132	1
4 oz.	3	158	3
4 oz.	5	210	16
4 oz.	5	246	14
4 oz.	3	297	20
4 oz.	3	229	13
4 oz.	8	221	16
4 oz.	9	298	20

*fish (cont.)

5	jack, canned	......
3	king, raw	......
5	Pacific, broiled	......
6	Spanish, broiled	......
5	mullet, striped, broiled	......
	perch	
7	freshwater, mixed species, broiled	......
4	ocean, broiled	......
	pike	
3	northern, broiled	......
5	walleye, raw	......
	pollock	
4	Atlantic, raw	......
6	walleye, broiled	......
	sticks (see fish, sticks)	
9	pompano, Florida, broiled	......
3	pout, ocean, raw	......
3	rockfish, Pacific, mixed species, broiled	......
23	roe, mixed species, raw	......
1	roughy, orange, raw	......
8	sablefish, smoked	......
	salmon	
4	Atlantic, raw	......
2	chinook, smoked	......

*See entry in Notes section for this class of food.

COMMON PORTION

AMOUNT	CSI	TOTAL CALORIES	TOTAL FAT GRAMS
4 oz.	5	176	7
4 oz.	3	118	2
4 oz.	5	?	?
4 oz.	6	178	7
4 oz.	5	169	5
4 oz.	7	132	1
4 oz.	4	137	2
4 oz.	3	128	1
4 oz.	5	105	1
4 oz.	4	104	1
4 oz.	6	128	1
4 oz.	9	238	14
4 oz.	3	89	1
4 oz.	3	137	1
4 oz.	23	158	7
4 oz.	1	142	8
4 oz.	8	290	23
4 oz.	4	77	7
4 oz.	2	132	5

*fish (cont.)

CSI	
4	chum, canned ....
4	coho, steamed..
8	loaf, typical ....
7	mousse, typical..
4	pink, raw ....
	sockeye
7	broiled..
4	canned..
	sardines
10	Atlantic, canned in oil, drained ....
5	Pacific, canned in tomato sauce ....
4	sashimi (raw tuna) ....
6	sea trout, mixed species, raw ....
	shark, mixed species
4	raw...
7	oil-egg-milk batter, pan-fried ....
6	smelt, rainbow, broiled................................
3	snapper, broiled..
10	sticks, from frozen pollock, breaded with egg and milk, fried............................
4	sunfish, pumpkinseed, raw ....
4	swordfish, broiled ....
	trout
5	mixed species, raw ....

*See entry in Notes section for this class of food.

COMMON PORTION

AMOUNT	CSI	TOTAL CALORIES	TOTAL FAT GRAMS
4 oz.	4	160	6
4 oz.	4	209	9
4 oz.	8	212	11
4 oz.	7	272	24
4 oz.	4	132	4
4 oz.	7	243	12
4 oz.	4	173	8
3 oz.	10	236	13
3 oz.	5	202	14
4 oz.	4	163	5
4 oz.	6	117	4
4 oz.	4	148	5
4 oz.	7	258	16
4 oz.	6	141	4
4 oz.	3	145	2
4 oz.	10	308	14
4 oz.	4	101	1
4 oz.	4	176	6
4 oz.	5	168	7

	*fish (cont.)
5	rainbow, broiled ....
	tuna
5	bluefin, broiled...
3	light, canned in soybean oil, drained.......
3	skipjack, fresh, raw....................................
3	white, canned in water ....
3	yellowfin, raw ....
	noodle casserole (see casserole)
	turbot (see flatfish)
	walleye (see pike or pollock)
2	whitefish, mixed species, smoked ....
5	whiting, mixed species, broiled....................
2	wolffish, Atlantic, raw.................................
	flour (see footnote 3, page 17)
	frankfurter
17	beef..
15	beef and pork..
12	chicken..
13	corn dog or pronto pup...............................
12	turkey..
	French fried potatoes (see vegetable, potato)
	French toast (see toast, French)
4	**frijoles** with cheese (cheese 6%).....................
	frosting (see cake)

*See entry in Notes section for this class of food.

68

COMMON PORTION

AMOUNT	CSI	TOTAL CALORIES	TOTAL FAT GRAMS
4 oz.	5	172	5
4 oz.	5	209	7
4 oz.	3	213	9
4 oz.	3	117	1
4 oz.	3	154	3
4 oz.	3	122	1
4 oz.	2	122	1
4 oz.	5	130	2
4 oz.	2	109	3
1 frank	7	180	16
1 frank	6	144	13
1 frank	5	116	9
one	13	344	28
1 frank	5	100	8
8 oz., cup	6	225	8

fruit (see footnote 3, page 17)
fruitcake (see cake)
fudge (see candy)
0   **Fudgesicle** ....

-G-

0   **gelatin dessert**, all flavors..............................
     gingersnaps (see cookies)
5   **goat**, wild, roasted...
11   **goose**, domesticated, roasted............................
     granola (see cereal)
     gravy
       cream, for chicken
1   made with skim milk, defatted.................
4   made with whole milk, defatted..............
2   turkey, defatted...
2   **guacamole**...

-H-

*ham
  cured, extra lean

COMMON PORTION

AMOUNT	CSI	TOTAL CALORIES	TOTAL FAT GRAMS
one	0	91	0
1 cup	0	142	0
4 oz.	5	162	3
4 oz.	11	270	14
¼ cup	1	39	2
¼ cup	2	55	4
¼ cup	1	28	2
¼ cup	1	62	5

	*ham (cont.)
5	roasted...
4	roasted, canned................................
	fresh
10	rump half, roasted............................
9	shank half, roasted...........................
17	patties, fully grilled, fresh and canned.........
	whole (arm picnics and hams), cured,
	purchased cooked
5	roasted...
5	unheated...
	hamburger patty
9	10% fat..
12	15% fat..
15	20% fat..
16	25% fat..
7	**hash** corned beef..............................
10	**head cheese** ....
0	**honey**...
4	**honey loaf**, pork and beef....................
7	**horsemeat** ....
0	**horseradish**..................................
	hot chocolate (see milk, cocoa)
1	**hummus** (olive oil 5%, tahini 5%).............
14	**hush puppies** (milk 27%, egg 17%)...........

*See entry in Notes section for this class of food.

COMMON PORTION

AMOUNT	CSI	TOTAL CALORIES	TOTAL FAT GRAMS
4 oz.	5	164	6
4 oz.	4	154	6
4 oz.	10	249	12
4 oz.	9	243	12
4 oz.	17	388	35
4 oz.	5	177	6
4 oz.	5	126	5
4 oz.	9	227	9
4 oz.	12	287	17
4 oz.	15	328	21
4 oz.	16	371	27
1 cup	15	400	25
2 oz.	5	120	9
1 tblsp.	0	64	0
2 oz.	2	72	3
4 oz.	7	177	7
1 tblsp.	0	6	0
4 oz.	1	194	10
5 pieces	9	256	12

-I-

ice cream

10	store brands (10% fat).....................................
15	rich (12% fat) ....
12	French vanilla soft serve...............................
5	**ice milk** (light ice cream)...............................
3	soft serve...

instant breakfast, all flavors

0	made with skim milk ....
3	made with whole milk ....

-J,K-

2	**jam or jelly**, typical...
	jelly roll (see cake)
	Jell-O (see gelatin dessert)
2	**ketchup** ....
15	**kielbasa** (kolbassy), pork and beef..................
15	**knackwurst** (knockworst), pork and beef.......
	kolbassy (see kielbasa)

COMMON PORTION

AMOUNT	CSI	TOTAL CALORIES	TOTAL FAT GRAMS
1 cup	**15**	329	18
1 cup	**19**	480	19
1 cup	**21**	317	23
1 cup	**6**	236	8
1 cup	**4**	224	5
1 cup	**1**	215	1
1 cup	**7**	279	9
1 tblsp.	**0**	55	0
1 tblsp.	**0**	0	0
2 oz.	**8**	177	16
2 oz.	**7**	174	16

-L-

*lamb
    brain
119   braised...
148   pan-fried ....
9   chop, loin, broiled.................................
18   heart, braised ....
33   kidneys, braised ....
    leg
8   shank half, choice, roasted.......................
9   sirloin half, choice, roasted.....................
    leg and shoulder, cubed for stew or kabob
10   braised...
8   broiled...
    liver
32   braised...
34   pan-fried ....
9   loin, choice, broiled or roasted...................
    New Zealand
10   rib, frozen, roasted...................................
9   leg, whole (shank and sirloin), roasted....
11   loin, broiled...
31   pancreas, braised...
10   rib, choice, broiled or roasted.......................

*See entry in Notes section for this class of food.

COMMON PORTION

AMOUNT	CSI	TOTAL CALORIES	TOTAL FAT GRAMS
4 oz.	**119**	165	11
4 oz.	**148**	309	25
4 oz.	**9**	245	10
4 oz.	**18**	210	9
4 oz.	**33**	156	4
4 oz.	**8**	203	8
4 oz.	**9**	230	10
4 oz.	**10**	253	10
4 oz.	**8**	210	8
4 oz.	**32**	249	10
4 oz.	**34**	269	14
4 oz.	**9**	235	11
4 oz.	**10**	222	11
4 oz.	**9**	205	8
4 oz.	**11**	226	9
4 oz.	**31**	263	15
4 oz.	**10**	266	15

	*lamb (cont.)
	shoulder
	(arm), choice
13	braised...
9	broiled or roasted.......................................
	(blade), choice
14	braised..
10	broiled or roasted.................................
20	tongue, braised ....
44	lard, pork ....
7	lasagna (see footnote 3, page 17)
	lasagna with meat sauce.................................
3	lefse type potato pancakes ....
10	liqueur, Irish cream ....
	liver (see beef, pork, chicken, etc.)
	liver paté (see paté)
21	liverwurst, pork.....................................
	loaf, meat or salmon
	(see meat loaf or salmon loaf)
4	lobster, spiny, mixed species, raw ....
4	lobster, northern, steamed................................
	London broil (see beef, round, top round)
	luxury loaf (see pork, luxury loaf)

*See entry in Notes section for this class of food.

COMMON PORTION

AMOUNT	CSI	TOTAL CALORIES	TOTAL FAT GRAMS
4 oz.	13	315	16
4 oz.	9	222	10
4 oz.	14	326	19
4 oz.	10	237	13
4 oz.	20	311	23
2 tblsp.	11	231	26
4 oz.	7	188	9
3 oz.	2	174	7
1 oz.	3	92	2
2 oz.	10	184	16
4 oz.	4	127	2
4 oz.	4	111	1

-M-

macaroni (see footnote 3, page 17)
macaroni
  cheese

7	from mix
4	homemade with 2% milk
4	with mayonnaise

  *margarine

8	imitation ("spread"), usually tub
16	liquid, stick, or soft

  marshmallows

12	chocolate covered
0	plain

  *mayonnaise (see under salad dressing)
meat (see beef, pork, lamb, etc.)
meat loaf

4	low-fat (10%) ground beef, egg white
10	typical
10	**meatballs**, Swedish

  milk

1	1% fat (low-fat)
2	2% fat (low-fat)
3	3.3% fat (whole milk)
3	3.7% fat

*See entry in Notes section for this class of food.

COMMON PORTION

AMOUNT	CSI	TOTAL CALORIES	TOTAL FAT GRAMS
1 cup	6	401	18
1 cup	12	336	19
1 cup	7	510	36
1 tblsp.	1	70	7
1 tblsp.	2	90	10
1 oz.	3	145	6
1 oz.	0	80	0
4 oz.	4	142	4
4 oz.	10	223	14
4 oz.	10	248	18
8 fl. oz.	2	102	3
8 fl. oz.	4	122	5
8 fl. oz.	7	149	8
8 fl. oz.	7	162	9

milk (cont.)
  buttermilk

1	skim milk (0.15% fat).............................
1	1% fat..
3	carob powder mix, 3 tsp. 8 oz. whole milk.
3	chocolate, chocolate syrup, 2 tblsp. in 8 oz. whole milk ....

  chocolate flavored

1	1% fat milk (commercial)........................
2	2% fat milk (commercial)........................
3	made from whole milk (commercial).......

  chocolate

3	powder mix, 2 to 3 heaping tsp. in 8 oz. whole milk.....................................
3	malted flavor mix, 3 heaping tsp. in 8 oz. whole milk ....

  cocoa or hot chocolate:

1	made with skim milk ....
3	made with whole milk ....
0	made with water, 1 tsp., 6 oz. water.......

  coconut milk (see nut, coconut)

11	condensed, canned, sweetened.....................

  evaporated

0	skimmed, canned ....
7	whole, canned ....

COMMON PORTION

AMOUNT	CSI	TOTAL CALORIES	TOTAL FAT GRAMS
8 fl. oz.	0	90	1
8 fl. oz.	2	98	2
8 fl. oz.	7	195	8
8 fl. oz.	7	232	9
8 fl. oz.	2	158	3
8 fl. oz.	4	194	7
8 fl. oz.	7	208	9
8 fl. oz.	7	226	9
8 fl. oz.	7	229	9
8 fl. oz.	2	154	2
8 fl. oz.	7	218	9
8 fl. oz.	1	137	1
1 fl. oz.	3	123	3
1 fl. oz.	0	25	0
1 fl. oz.	2	42	2

	milk (cont.)
4	goat ....
	ice (see ice milk)
3	malted (no chocolate), 3 heaping tsp. in 8 oz. whole milk ....
	shake
3	all flavors (most fast food and other restaurants)...
9	all flavors, specialty ice cream stores......
0	skim ....
0	soy...
	milk shake (see milk, shake)
5	**mix**, trail, commercial (peanuts, sunflower seeds, raisins, carob) ....
5	**moose**, roasted ....
14	**mortadella**, beef and pork.............................
	mousse, chocolate or salmon (see pie, chocolate; fish, salmon; pudding)
	muffin
	English
5	with butter...
0	plain ....
4	oatmeal raisin, typical ....
4	plain, typical..

COMMON PORTION

AMOUNT	CSI	TOTAL CALORIES	TOTAL FAT GRAMS
8 fl. oz.	**8**	168	10
8 fl. oz.	**8**	236	10
16 fl. oz.	**8**	442	11
16 fl. oz.	**32**	671	39
8 fl. oz.	**0**	85	0
8 fl. oz.	**0**	79	5
½ cup	**3**	352	20
4 oz.	**5**	152	1
2 oz.	**7**	178	14
1	**3**	186	5
1	**0**	133	1
3 oz.	**3**	229	8
3 oz.	**3**	195	8

mussels (see shellfish)
2   **mustard**..

-N-

9   **nachos** with cheese (cheese 15%) ....
noodles
5   Chinese, chow mein (wheat, flour,
             hydrogenated vegetable oil) ....
2   egg, cooked ....
nuts
     almonds
6   dried, blanched or unblanched...................
6   oil roasted or toasted, blanched or
                 unblanched.......................................
7   beechnuts, dried ....
19   Brazil, dried, unblanched ....
1   butternuts, dried ....
     cashew
10   dry roasted..
11   oil roasted...
     chestnuts
       Chinese
0   boiled and steamed...............................

86

COMMON PORTION

AMOUNT	CSI	TOTAL CALORIES	TOTAL FAT GRAMS
1 tblsp.	0	11	1
4 oz.	9	233	7
1 cup	2	237	14
4 oz.	2	152	2
1 oz.	1	166	15
1 oz.	2	171	15
1 oz.	2	164	14
1 oz.	5	186	19
1 oz.	0	174	16
1 oz.	3	163	13
1 oz.	3	163	14
1 oz.	0	44	0

CSI 4 oz.	
	nuts (cont.)
0	roasted..
0	European, roasted...............................
0	boiled and roasted..............................
0	Japanese, boiled and steamed ....
0	dried..
0	roasted..
	coconut
	meat
67	dried..
32	dried, flaked, canned ....
36	shredded...
48	toasted..
34	raw ....
70	whipped to shortening-like cream ....
35	"cream" raw.......................................
18	"cream" canned...................................
24	"milk" raw ....
22	"milk" canned.....................................
0	"water" ....
	filberts (see nuts, hazelnuts)
	ginkgo
0	canned..
0	dried..
	hazelnuts or filberts

COMMON PORTION

AMOUNT	CSI	TOTAL CALORIES	TOTAL FAT GRAMS
1 oz.	0	68	0
1 oz.	0	70	1
1 oz.	0	37	0
1 oz.	0	16	0
1 oz.	0	102	0
1 oz.	0	57	0
1 oz.	17	191	19
1 oz.	8	126	9
1 oz.	9	142	10
1 oz.	12	168	13
1 oz.	9	100	9
1 oz.	18	194	20
1 oz.	9	94	10
1 oz.	4	54	5
1 oz.	6	65	7
1 oz.	5	56	6
1 oz.	0	5	0
1 oz.	0	32	0
1 oz.	0	99	1

nuts (cont.)

6	dried, blanched or unblanched..................
6	unblanched, dry or oil roasted.................
8	hickory, dried ....
13	macadamia, oil roasted or dried ....
8	mixed (cashews, almonds, peanuts, hazelnuts, pecans), dry roasted ....
8	peanuts, all types, dry or oil roasted ....
6	pecans, oil roasted or dry roasted or dried .
36	pilinuts-canarytree, dried ....
11	pine, piñon, dried................................
8	pistachio, dry roasted...........................
4	soybean kernels, roasted or toasted.............
	walnuts
4	black, dried................................
6	English or Persian, dried.......................

-O-

17	**octopus** (see footnote 1, page 17) ....
	***oil**
99	avocado..
8	canola..
97	coconut ....

*See entry in Notes section for this class of food.

COMMON PORTION

AMOUNT	CSI	TOTAL CALORIES	TOTAL FAT GRAMS
1 oz.	1	189	19
1 oz.	1	188	19
1 oz.	2	187	18
1 oz.	3	202	20
1 oz.	2	169	15
1 oz.	2	164	14
1 oz.	2	191	19
1 oz.	9	204	23
1 oz.	3	161	17
1 oz.	2	172	15
1 oz.	1	129	7
1 oz.	1	172	16
1 oz.	2	182	18
3 oz.	13	93	1
1 tblsp.	2	126	14
1 tblsp.	1	126	14
1 tblsp.	12	126	14

	*oil (cont.)
14	corn ....
29	cottonseed ....
15	olive ....
55	palm ....
91	palm kernel ....
19	peanut ....
10	safflower ....
16	sesame..
16	soybean ....
15	sunflower, hydrogenated ....
11	sunflower, nonhydrogenated..............................
	olive loaf (see pork)
1	**olives**, green, pickled.......................................
1	**olives**, Sevillano/Ascolano, ripe, pitted, "small" and "large" ....
1	**olives**, Sevillano/Ascolano, ripe, pitted, "jumbo" ....
1	**olives**, Sevillano/Ascolano, ripe, pitted, "super colossal" ....
	omelet (see eggs)
	onion rings (see vegetable, onion, rings)
	oysters (see shellfish)
	oyster stew (see soup, oyster stew)
	oxtails (see beef)

*See entry in Notes section for this class of food.

COMMON PORTION

AMOUNT	CSI	TOTAL CALORIES	TOTAL FAT GRAMS
1 tblsp.	2	126	14
1 tblsp.	4	120	14
1 tblsp.	2	119	14
1 tblsp.	7	126	14
1 tblsp.	11	120	14
1 tblsp.	2	120	14
1 tblsp.	1	120	14
1 tblsp.	2	120	14
1 tblsp.	2	120	14
1 tblsp.	2	120	14
1 tblsp.	1	120	14
3 large	0	13	1
3 olives	0	13	1
3 olives	0	21	2
3 olives	0	36	3

-P-

pancakes

6	cornmeal, typical...
12	potato (eggs 12%, margarine 7%)...............
1	modified breakfast, with oil and skim milk, no egg yolks ....
	typical breakfast
4	with butter and syrup.............................
7	plain ....
0	*pasta** (see footnote 3, page 17)......................
3	**paste**, almond...

pastrami

18	beef ....
5	turkey ....

pastry, Danish

8	cheese ....
6	cinnamon ....
5	fruit ....
23	**paté**, liver..
8	**Pavlova**, berry, typical ....
11	**peanut butter**, smooth or chunky style (contains added fat)...............................

peanuts (see nuts or candy)

peanut oil (see oil)

*See entry in Notes section for this class of food.

94

COMMON PORTION

AMOUNT	CSI	TOTAL CALORIES	TOTAL FAT GRAMS
5 oz.	7	228	7
5 oz.	15	945	24
5 oz.	1	212	6
8 oz.	9	520	14
5 oz.	8	258	10
1 cup	0	25	0
1 oz.	1	127	8
2 oz.	9	198	17
2 oz.	5	80	3
3 oz.	6	330	23
3 oz.	5	337	16
3 oz.	4	303	14
2 oz.	12	120	10
4 oz.	8	227	10
1 tblsp.	2	94	8

5	**peppered loaf**, pork and beef ....
11	**pheasant** (see footnote 1, page 17) ....
	pickle and pimento loaf (see pork, pickle and pimento loaf)
	pie
13	banana cream, single crust (see footnote 5, page 18)...............................
3	Boston cream, homemade ....
	chocolate cream
14	single crust (see footnote 5, page 18) .....
12	mousse (see footnote 5, page 18) ....
16	coconut cream, single crust (see footnote 5, page 18)...............................
	crust only
18	made with lard (see footnote 5, page 18).
23	chocolate crumb (see footnote 5, page 18)...............................
17	commercial (see footnote 5, page 18)......
15	graham cracker, commercial (see footnote 5, page 18) ....
7	made with oil (see footnote 5, page 18).
14	made with shortening (see footnote 5, page 18)...............................
23	made with whole eggs (see footnote 5, page 18)...............................

COMMON PORTION

AMOUNT	CSI	TOTAL CALORIES	TOTAL FAT GRAMS
2 oz.	3	84	4
4 oz.	11	241	11
⅛ pie	9	335	20
⅛ pie	2	210	6
⅛ pie	17	368	23
⅛ pie	10	249	15
⅛ pie	19	341	22
⅛ pie	4	129	9
⅛ pie	5	149	12
⅛ pie	4	130	9
⅛ pie	5	178	11
⅛ pie	2	138	9
⅛ pie	3	142	11
⅛ pie	6	159	11

pie (cont.)

11	custard, single crust (see footnote 5, page 18)..
7	fruit, double crust (see footnote 5, page 18).
14	grasshopper, single crumb crust (see footnote 5, page 18)..........................
9	lemon meringue, single crust (see footnote 5, page 18)......................................
5	mincemeat, single crust (see footnote 5, page 18)...
10	pan-fried, fruit (snack type)..........................
11	pecan, single crust (see footnote 5, page 18)
7	pumpkin, single crust (see footnote 5, page 18)..
	tamale (see tamale)
	zucchini (see vegetable, zucchini)

pie tart (see tart)

pig's feet or tail (see pork, feet or tail)

pimento loaf (see pork, pickle and pimento loaf)

pizza, thick crust

4	cheese (see footnote 2, page 17).....................
5	combination (see footnote 2, page 17) ....
3	pepperoni (see footnote 2, page 17) ....

COMMON PORTION

AMOUNT	CSI	TOTAL CALORIES	TOTAL FAT GRAMS
⅛ pie	11	259	14
⅛ pie	8	378	20
⅛ pie	17	431	26
⅛ pie	11	339	15
⅛ pie	5	248	10
1	7	266	14
⅛ pie	11	512	31
⅛ pic	11	314	14
¼ pie	11	664	16
¼ pie	17	842	33
¼ pie	10	674	19

pizza, thin crust (cont.)

2   pepper-mushroom-onion (see footnote 2, page 17)......................................

pizza, thin crust

7   cheese (see footnote 2, page 17).................

8   combination (see footnote 2, page 17)........

6   pepperoni (see footnote 2, page 17)............

3   pepper-mushroom-onion (see footnote 2, page 17)......................................

popcorn

    air popped

4   with 1 tsp. margarine ....

0   plain ....

20   commercially popped, plain or cheese-flavored...

5   caramel corn...

14 **popover** ....

0 **popsicle** ....

5 **Pop-Tart**...

*****pork**

147   brains, braised ....

20   chitterlings, simmered............................

    chop, rib

11   braised..

11   broiled..

*See entry in Notes section for this class of food.

COMMON PORTION

AMOUNT	CSI	TOTAL CALORIES	TOTAL FAT GRAMS
¼ pie	6	574	9
¼ pie	16	552	24
¼ pie	20	676	38
¼ pie	13	509	23
¼ pie	9	419	14
3 cups	1	105	5
3 cups	0	69	1
3 cups	5	116	5
3 cups	5	468	21
2 oz.	7	131	6
1	0	99	0
1	2	196	6
4 oz.	147	156	9
4 oz.	20	344	28
4 oz.	11	316	17
4 oz.	11	295	17

	*pork (cont.)
11	pan-fried ....
10	roasted..
	chop, with filet (see pork, loin, center loin)
	chop, without filet (see pork, loin, center rib)
	feet
12	cured and pickled ....
11	simmered ....
10	headcheese (cured meat)............................
14	heart, braised.....................................
29	kidneys, braised ....
22	liver, braised.....................................
20	liver cheese (cured meat)..........................
	liver sausage (see liverwurst)
	loin
	blade
15	braised..
14	broiled..
13	pan-fried or roasted ....
	center loin
12	braised..
12	pan-fried ....
10	broiled..
11	roasted..

*See entry in Notes section for this class of food.

COMMON PORTION

AMOUNT	CSI	TOTAL CALORIES	TOTAL FAT GRAMS
4 oz.	**11**	293	18
4 oz.	**10**	280	16
4 oz.	**12**	220	14
4 oz.	**11**	220	14
4 oz.	**10**	240	18
4 oz.	**14**	197	6
4 oz.	**29**	170	5
4 oz.	**22**	188	4
4 oz.	**20**	344	29
4 oz.	**15**	355	20
4 oz.	**14**	340	20
4 oz.	**13**	319	19
4 oz.	**12**	308	14
4 oz.	**12**	301	16
4 oz.	**10**	261	10
4 oz.	**11**	272	12

	*pork (cont.)
	center rib
11	braised...
11	broiled or pan-fried..............................
10	roasted...
	tenderloin or top loin (see below under their names)
23	lungs, braised ....
4	luxury loaf (cured meat) ....
9	olive loaf (cured meat)...............................
11	pickle and pimento loaf (cured meat)..........
25	rinds ....
	roast (see pork, loin, center rib)
10	rump, roasted ....
	salami (see salami)
	sausage (see sausage)
9	shank, roasted...
11	shoulder, arm picnic, braised or roasted......
13	shoulder, blade, Boston, braised ....
13	shoulder, blade, Boston, broiled or roasted.
	sirloin
11	braised or broiled.......................................
10	roasted..
20	spareribs, lean and fat, braised ....
22	tail, simmered...

*See entry in Notes section for this class of food.

COMMON PORTION

AMOUNT	CSI	TOTAL CALORIES	TOTAL FAT GRAMS
4 oz.	11	315	14
4 oz.	11	292	15
4 oz.	10	277	14
4 oz.	23	112	3
2 oz.	2	80	2
2 oz.	4	134	10
2 oz.	6	148	12
2 cups	5	150	9
4 oz.	11	271	12
4 oz.	10	251	12
4 oz.	9	244	12
4 oz.	14	333	17
4 oz.	13	300	17
4 oz.	11	285	13
4 oz.	10	268	12
4 oz.	20	451	29
4 oz.	22	449	41

	*pork (cont.)
7	tenderloin, roasted...
16	tongue, braised ....
11	top loin, braised or broiled or pan-fried......
	pork rinds (see pork, rinds)
	potato chips (see chips)
	potato, French fries (see vegetable, potato)
	potato pancakes (see pancakes, potato)
	potato (see vegetable, potato)
	potato sticks (see vegetable, potato, sticks)
	pretzels
3	twists..
3	sticks ....
	pronto pup (see frankfurter)
	*pudding
	all flavors, dessert type
0	from mix, made with skim milk ....
3	from mix, made with whole milk............
3	banana cream ....
28	Bavarian cream ....
	blood (see blood pudding)
7	bread, homemade, typical.............................
3	butterscotch...
17	chiffon, all flavors ....

*See entry in Notes section for this class of food.

AMOUNT	CSI	TOTAL CALORIES	TOTAL FAT GRAMS
4 oz.	7	188	5
4 oz.	16	307	21
4 oz.	11	304	15
5	0	39	1
1 cup	0	39	1
1 cup	1	251	1
1 cup	6	307	8
1 cup	7	330	9
1 cup	37	388	35
1 cup	16	441	16
1 cup	7	328	9
1 cup	25	414	12

	*pudding (cont.)
3	chocolate..
	chocolate
3	fudge..
15	soufflé...
6	mousse ....
4	coconut cream ....
6	corn ....
2	lemon, homemade.................................
15	plum..
3	rice, plain ....
9	tapioca, homemade ....

-Q-

quiche (see vegetable, broccoli)

-R-

rabbit

6	domesticated, composite of cuts, roasted.....
8	domesticated, composite of cuts, stewed .....
8	wild, composite of cuts, stewed ....

*See entry in Notes section for this class of food.

COMMON PORTION

AMOUNT	CSI	TOTAL CALORIES	TOTAL FAT GRAMS
1 cup	6	352	9
1 cup	7	348	9
1 cup	8	127	8
1 cup	9	380	31
1 cup	11	356	13
1 cup	13	280	14
1 cup	4	114	2
1 cup	30	895	47
1 cup	7	365	11
1 cup	15	255	9
4 oz.	6	174	7
4 oz.	8	233	10
4 oz.	8	196	4

ravioli

2	cheese, canned ....
2	meat, canned ....
10	meat, homemade ....
9	cheese, homemade ....
20	**relleno**, chile ....

rice

8	fried..
9	green ....
2	pilaf...
0	Spanish ....

rinds, pork (see pork, rinds)

roe (see fish, roe)

roll

cabbage (see cabbage roll)

12	crescent ....
14	sticky nut...
8	sweet, cinnamon...

(see also under generic names like
"brioche" or "croissant")

17	**rumaki** (chopped liver rolled in bacon)..........

COMMON PORTION

AMOUNT	CSI	TOTAL CALORIES	TOTAL FAT GRAMS
8 oz.	4	233	5
8 oz.	4	244	7
8 oz.	20	460	30
8 oz.	17	374	10
1 chile	19	267	21
1 cup	18	338	14
1 cup	15	299	16
1 cup	4	365	16
1 cup	1	195	3
1 oz.	3	101	3
3 oz.	11	370	17
one 4-inch	5	276	11
1 piece	2	23	1

-S-

salad

2	aspic, with mayonnaise, crab, asparagus......
2	Athene, typical ....
6	carrot raisin, typical..
	*chef's
9	egg, cheese, ham, turkey, ½ cup Thousand Island dressing ....
7	as above, but low-calorie Thousand Island dressing..
5	as above, but low-calorie Thousand Island dressing, no egg.............................
9	chicken, with mayonnaise ....
25	egg, with mayonnaise.....................................
5	fruit, with marshmallows and whipped cream ....
4	macaroni, with mayonnaise............................
5	potato, typical..
3	tabouli, typical ....
8	taco, typical...
3	three bean..
	tuna
4	with light mayonnaise ....
6	with regular mayonnaise ....

*See entry in Notes section for this class of food.

COMMON PORTION

AMOUNT	CSI	TOTAL CALORIES	TOTAL FAT GRAMS
1 cup	**3**	162	12
1 cup	**3**	195	14
1 cup	**6**	152	9
1 salad	**40**	910	67
1 salad	**31**	624	40
1 salad	**19**	545	34
½ cup	**9**	353	32
½ cup	**24**	252	23
1 cup	**7**	180	9
1 cup	**7**	510	36
1 cup	**10**	392	26
1 cup	**3**	269	19
1 cup	**8**	168	13
1 cup	**4**	287	23
½ cup	**4**	196	15
½ cup	**5**	272	25

	salad (cont.)
4	Waldorf ....
	salad dressing
11	blue cheese..
4	low-calorie..
11	French...
1	low-calorie..
8	Italian...
2	low-calorie..
17	*mayonnaise..
5	light mayonnaise (see footnote 4, page 18)...
6	imitation, soy oil...................................
16	imitation, soy oil, commercial..............
11	oil (olive oil 2 tblsp.) and vinegar (2 tblsp.).
10	ranch type..
1	with skim milk or buttermilk or nonfat yogurt...
8	Russian ....
3	low-calorie..
2	Thousand Island...
4	low-calorie..
	salami
7	beef, cooked...

*See entry in Notes section for this class of food.

114

COMMON PORTION

AMOUNT	CSI	TOTAL CALORIES	TOTAL FAT GRAMS
1 cup	6	382	36
2 tblsp.	3	147	16
2 tblsp.	1	23	2
2 tblsp.	3	134	13
2 tblsp.	1	44	2
2 tblsp.	1	90	8
2 tblsp.	1	32	3
2 tblsp.	4	200	22
2 tblsp.	2	90	10
2 tblsp.	1	69	6
2 tblsp.	4	198	22
2 tblsp.	2	121	13
2 tblsp.	3	107	3
2 tblsp.	0	14	0
2 tblsp.	1	90	6
2 tblsp.	1	46	2
2 tblsp.	2	120	2
2 tblsp.	1	49	4
1 oz.	2	37	3

	salami (cont.)
13	beef and pork, cooked.....................................
	beerwurst
18	beef ....
10	pork ....
18	Genoa (hard) ....
8	turkey, cooked...
	salmon loaf (see fish, salmon, loaf)
	salmon mousse (see fish, salmon, mousse)
0	salsa..
	sashimi (see fish)
	sauce
0	barbecue...
	béarnaise (see sauce, hollandaise)
0	butterscotch flavored.................................
3	caramel, homemade ....
0	caramel flavored ....
11	cheese ....
2	cheese (low-fat cheese) ....
10	chocolate, fudge type.................................
15	custard..
	hollandaise or béarnaise
23	with butterfat, from mix............................
6	with vegetable oil, from mix ....
0	marinara, canned.......................................

COMMON PORTION

AMOUNT	CSI	TOTAL CALORIES	TOTAL FAT GRAMS
1 oz.	3	70	6
1 oz.	5	94	9
1 oz.	3	57	4
1 oz.	5	115	10
1 oz.	2	51	3
¼ cup	0	24	0
1 oz.	0	21	1
¼ cup	0	264	0
¼ cup	2	291	7
¼ cup	0	264	0
¼ cup	6	133	11
¼ cup	1	52	3
¼ cup	7	251	10
¼ cup	9	93	5
1 oz.	6	78	8
1 oz.	2	26	2
¼ cup	0	43	2

	sauce (cont.)
	Italian
1	meatless ....
5	with meat..
3	mushroom, from mix.......................................
8	sour cream, from mix.....................................
0	soy...
1	spaghetti, meatless, canned ....
3	Stroganoff, from mix ....
12	tartar...
0	teriyaki, bottled ....
0	tomato, canned ....
5	white ....
	sausage
17	beef, smoked, canned.....................................
	blood (see blood pudding)
7	honey roll, beef..
15	Italian, pork, cooked.....................................
16	Polish ....
17	pork, link, smoked..
	pork liver (see liverwurst)
19	pork and beef, smoked, link..........................
17	pork (may be called "country style"), fresh, cooked..
11	turkey, cooked..

COMMON PORTION

AMOUNT	CSI	TOTAL CALORIES	TOTAL FAT GRAMS
¼ cup	0	42	2
¼ cup	3	82	5
1 oz.	1	24	1
1 oz.	2	47	3
2 tblsp.	0	7	0
¼ cup	0	68	3
2 tblsp.	0	13	1
1 oz.	3	305	33
2 tblsp.	0	12	0
¼ cup	0	19	0
¼ cup	3	101	8
2 oz.	4	181	15
2 oz.	4	104	6
2 oz.	7	183	15
2 oz.	8	187	16
2 oz.	8	221	18
2 oz.	10	191	17
2 oz.	9	209	18
2 oz.	5	122	8

sausage (cont.)

14   Vienna (beef and pork), canned ....

scallops (see shellfish)

12   **scone** ....

seeds

11   cottonseed kernels (glandless), roasted ....

pumpkin and squash

10   kernels, dried or roasted ....

4   whole, roasted ....

4   safflower, kernels, dried ....

sesame

8   whole, roasted and toasted ....

8   kernels, decorticated, dried ....

7   kernels, decorticated, toasted ....

squash (see seeds, pumpkin)

sunflower, kernels

6   dried or dry roasted ....

7   toasted or oil roasted ....

11   watermelon, dried ....

shake, milk (see milk)

*shellfish

7   abalone, mixed species, pan-fried ....

clams, mixed species

7   breaded and pan-fried (egg 5%, milk 1%).

4   canned ....

*See entry in Notes section for this class of food.

COMMON PORTION

AMOUNT	CSI	TOTAL CALORIES	TOTAL FAT GRAMS
2 oz.	7	160	14
one 4-inch	6	294	12
1 oz.	3	143	10
1 oz.	2	151	13
1 oz.	1	127	6
1 oz.	1	147	11
1 oz.	2	161	14
1 oz.	2	167	16
1 oz.	2	161	14
1 oz.	1	164	14
1 oz.	2	176	16
1 oz.	3	158	14
3 oz.	5	161	6
3 oz.	5	171	9
3 oz.	3	126	2

	*shellfish (cont.)
4	steamed..
2	raw ....
	conch: closely resembles whelk in fat type and content
4	steamers ....
	mussels, blue
2	raw ....
4	steamed ....
	oysters, eastern
8	breaded and pan-fried (egg 5%, milk 1%).
4	raw, fresh or canned....................................
8	steamed ....
14	Rockefeller ....
	scallops
3	broiled..
7	mixed species, breaded and pan-fried (egg 5%, milk 1%)...............................
7	whelk, steamed...
2	**sherbet**, fruit flavored................................
	shortening
26	made from soybean oil.................................
32	made from soybean and palm oils...............
	shrimp
	mixed species

*See entry in Notes section for this class of food.

COMMON PORTION

AMOUNT	CSI	TOTAL CALORIES	TOTAL FAT GRAMS
3 oz.	3	126	2
3 oz.	2	63	1
3 oz.	3	126	2
3 oz.	2	97	3
3 oz.	3	196	5
6 medium	6	222	14
6 medium	3	77	3
6 medium	3	235	6
6 oysters	20	324	24
3 oz.	2	96	1
3 oz.	7	244	12
3 oz.	6	233	1
1 cup	3	270	4
1 tblsp.	3	113	13
1 tblsp.	4	113	13

shrimp (cont.)

12	breaded and pan-fried (egg 5%, milk 1%).
11	steamed...

Louis

2	no egg, ½ cup low-calorie Thousand Island dressing..................................
5	with egg, ½ cup low-calorie Thousand Island dressing..................................
6	with egg, ½ cup Thousand Island dressing...
0	**sorbet** ....

***soup**

asparagus, cream of

1	condensed, prepared with water ....
2	condensed, prepared with milk.................

bean, black

0	condensed, prepared with water ....
2	with ham, chunky, canned, ready to serve.
1	with bacon, condensed, prepared with water ....
1	with frankfurters, condensed, prepared with water......................................
0	broth, beef or chicken ....
1	Scotch, condensed, prepared with water..

*See entry in Notes section for this class of food.

COMMON PORTION

AMOUNT	CSI	TOTAL CALORIES	TOTAL FAT GRAMS
4 oz.	**12**	274	14
4 oz.	**11**	112	1
1 salad	**10**	364	17
1 salad	**22**	443	23
1 salad	**28**	730	50
1 cup	**0**	255	0
1 cup	**1**	87	4
1 cup	**2**	166	8
1 cup	**0**	116	2
1 cup	**2**	231	9
1 cup	**1**	173	6
1 cup	**1**	187	7
1 cup	**0**	16	1
1 cup	**1**	80	3

	*soup (cont.)
	beef
2	chunky, canned, ready-to-serve.................
1	mushroom, prepared with water..............
1	noodle, condensed, prepared with water..
6	beer-cheese ....
	bouillon (see broth, beef or chicken)
	celery, cream of, condensed
3	prepared with milk ....
1	prepared with water....................................
	cheese, condensed
5	prepared with milk ....
4	prepared with water....................................
	chicken
0	broth, condensed, prepared with water ....
2	chunky, canned, ready to serve ....
	cream of
1	condensed, prepared with water ....
3	condensed, prepared with milk................
3	dumplings, condensed, prepared with water.
0	gumbo, condensed, prepared with water......
1	mushroom, condensed, prepared with water
	noodle
1	chunky, canned, ready to serve ....
0	condensed, prepared with water ....

*See entry in Notes section for this class of food.

AMOUNT	CSI	TOTAL CALORIES	TOTAL FAT GRAMS
1 cup	2	171	5
1 cup	1	?	3
1 cup	1	84	3
1 cup	14	308	23
1 cup	3	165	10
1 cup	1	90	6
1 cup	5	230	15
1 cup	4	155	11
1 cup	0	39	1
1 cup	2	178	7
1 cup	1	116	7
1 cup	3	191	12
1 cup	3	97	6
1 cup	0	56	1
1 cup	1	?	9
1 cup	1	?	6
1 cup	0	75	3

*soup (cont.)

1	with meatballs, canned, ready to serve....

rice

1	chunky, canned, ready to serve ....
0	condensed, prepared with water ....

vegetable

1	chunky, canned, ready to serve ....
1	condensed, prepared with water ....
2	chili, beef, condensed, prepared with water.

clam chowder, Manhattan, chunky

1	canned, ready to serve ....
0	condensed, prepared with water ....

clam chowder, New England

2	condensed, prepared with milk.................
0	condensed, prepared with water ....
0	consommé, plus gelatin, condensed, prepared with water...........................
0	crab, canned, ready to serve........................
3	egg drop ....
0	escarole, canned, ready to serve..................
0	gazpacho, canned, ready to serve................
2	hot and sour......................................
1	lentil with ham, canned, ready to serve ......

minestrone

1	chunky, canned, ready to serve ....

*See entry in Notes section for this class of food.

COMMON PORTION

AMOUNT	CSI	TOTAL CALORIES	TOTAL FAT GRAMS
1 cup	1	99	4
1 cup	1	127	3
1 cup	0	60	2
1 cup	1	167	5
1 cup	1	74	3
1 cup	2	169	7
1 cup	1	133	3
1 cup	0	78	2
1 cup	2	163	7
1 cup	0	95	3
1 cup	0	29	0
1 cup	0	76	2
1 cup	8	79	4
1 cup	0	27	2
1 cup	0	57	2
1 cup	5	124	6
1 cup	1	140	3
1 cup	1	127	3

***soup** (cont.)

0	condensed, prepared with water ....
	mushroom
	cream of, condensed
3	prepared with milk ....
1	prepared with water.............................
5	Hungarian ....
1	plus beef stock, condensed, prepared with water ....
0	barley, condensed, prepared with water ...
	onion, condensed
0	prepared with water.............................
3	cream of, prepared with milk..................
1	cream of, prepared with water.................
2	with cheese......................................
	oyster stew, condensed
3	prepared with milk ....
2	prepared with water.............................
	pea, green, condensed
2	prepared with milk ....
1	prepared with water.............................
	pea, split
1	plus ham, chunky, condensed, prepared with water.......................................
1	chunky, canned, ready to serve ....

*See entry in Notes section for this class of food.

COMMON PORTION

AMOUNT	CSI	TOTAL CALORIES	TOTAL FAT GRAMS
1 cup	**0**	83	3
1 cup	**3**	203	14
1 cup	**1**	129	9
1 cup	**12**	212	16
1 cup	**1**	85	4
1 cup	**0**	?	2
1 cup	**0**	57	2
1 cup	**3**	?	9
1 cup	**1**	?	5
1 cup	**4**	?	?
1 cup	**3**	134	8
1 cup	**2**	59	4
1 cup	**2**	239	7
1 cup	**1**	164	3
1 cup	**1**	189	4
1 cup	**1**	184	4

*soup (cont.)

1	pepper pot, condensed, prepared with water.
	potato, cream of, condensed
2	prepared with milk ....
1	prepared with water...................................
	Scotch broth (see broth, Scotch)
	shrimp, cream of, condensed
3	prepared with milk ....
2	prepared with water...................................
1	stockpot, condensed, prepared with water ...
	tomato
	condensed
2	prepared with milk ....
0	prepared with water...............................
1	beef plus noodle, condensed, prepared with water.......................................
	bisque, condensed
2	prepared with milk ....
0	prepared with water...............................
0	rice, condensed, prepared with water.......
	turkey
1	chunky, canned, ready to serve ....
0	noodle, condensed, prepared with water..
0	vegetable, condensed, prepared with water ....

*See entry in Notes section for this class of food.

COMMON PORTION

AMOUNT	CSI	TOTAL CALORIES	TOTAL FAT GRAMS
1 cup	1	103	5
1 cup	2	148	7
1 cup	1	73	2
1 cup	3	165	9
1 cup	2	90	5
1 cup	1	100	4
1 cup	2	160	6
1 cup	0	86	2
1 cup	1	140	4
1 cup	2	198	7
1 cup	0	123	3
1 cup	0	120	3
1 cup	1	136	4
1 cup	0	69	2
1 cup	0	74	3

	*soup (cont.)
1	turtle...
16	turtle, mock ....
	vegetable
0	chunky, canned, ready to serve ....
0	vegetarian, condensed, prepared with water ....
1	plus beef, condensed, prepared with water.
0	plus beef broth, condensed, prepared with water ....
	vichyssoise, condensed
2	prepared with milk ....
1	prepared with water....................................
	soy sauce (see sauce, soy)
	soybeans
1	boiled ....
4	roasted...
	spaghetti (see footnote 3, page 17)
3	spaghetti with meat sauce...............................
17	squid, mixed species, pan-fried.......................
6	squirrel, roasted ....
	steak (see various cuts under beef)
	stew
4	beef vegetable ....
	oyster (see soup, oyster stew)

*See entry in Notes section for this class of food.

COMMON PORTION

AMOUNT	CSI	TOTAL CALORIES	TOTAL FAT GRAMS
1 cup	**2**	92	4
1 cup	**34**	247	16
1 cup	**0**	122	4
1 cup	**0**	72	2
1 cup	**1**	79	2
1 cup	**0**	81	2
1 cup	**2**	148	7
1 cup	**1**	73	2
½ cup	**1**	149	8
½ cup	**3**	405	22
1 cup	**4**	237	7
4 oz.	**17**	199	8
4 oz.	**6**	154	4
1 cup	**8**	246	14

	*sundae
4	caramel ....
4	hot fudge ....
4	strawberry ....
	sunflower seeds or oil (see seeds or oil)
1	**syrup**, chocolate ....
	sweet potato (see vegetable, sweet potato)
	sweet roll (see roll)

-T-

2	**tabouli** ....
9	**taco** ....
	taco salad (see salad)
4	**tahini** ....
6	**tamale**, pie, typical...................................
	taro chips (see chips)
9	**tart**, pie, commercial................................
1	**tempeh** ....
13	**tempura** (6 prawns)...................................
	toast, French
2	made with skim milk, egg substitute...........
16	typical...
3	**tofu**, pan-fried...

*See entry in Notes section for this class of food.

COMMON PORTION

AMOUNT	CSI	TOTAL CALORIES	TOTAL FAT GRAMS
1 sundae	6	304	9
1 sundae	6	284	9
1 sundae	5	268	8
¼ cup	1	138	2
1 cup	3	269	19
6 oz.	14	369	21
1 tblsp.	1	85	8
1 cup	16	441	28
one	7	275	15
½ cup	1	165	6
4 oz.	13	249	13
2 slices	2	232	8
2 slices	10	262	12
1 oz.	1	65	6

Tofutti
0	lite-lite ....
2	made with vegetable oil...............................

topping (see cream, whipped)

tortilla
5	mix (enriched with lard) ....
8	flour, fried...

tostada
8	with cheese, beef and beans (cheese 9%, beef 7%)..
5	with cheese and beans (cheese 7%).............
5	with cheese and guacamole (avocado 33%, cheese 9%)...

trail mix (see mix)

tripe (see beef)

tuna casserole (see fish, tuna)

*turkey

all classes
8	dark meat, roasted ....
5	light meat, roasted ....
25	giblets, simmered..
14	gizzard, simmered.......................................
15	heart, simmered..
38	liver, simmered...
10	neck, simmered...

*See entry in Notes section for this class of food.

COMMON PORTION

AMOUNT	CSI	TOTAL CALORIES	TOTAL FAT GRAMS
1 cup	**0**	180	1
1 cup	**3**	420	24
⅓ cup	**2**	150	4
2 oz.	**4**	214	11
1 tostada	**15**	333	17
1 tostada	**7**	223	10
1 tostada	**12**	179	12
4 oz.	**8**	212	8
4 oz.	**5**	178	4
2 oz.	**13**	95	3
2 oz.	**7**	92	2
2 oz.	**7**	100	3
2 oz.	**19**	96	3
4 oz.	**10**	204	8

*turkey (cont.)

7	wing, roasted...
8	ground (includes flesh and skin from all classes)..
5	ham (cured thigh meat)...............................
5	roll, light and dark meat or light meat only.
	sausage (see sausage, turkey)
9	**turnover**, fruit, commercial ....

-V-

*veal

	chop (see veal, loin or, especially for restaurants, veal, rib)
9	cutlet, braised or broiled ....
9	ground, broiled...
12	heart, braised..
47	kidneys, braised ....
11	leg and shoulder, cubed for stew, braised ...
	leg (top round)
10	braised..
8	breaded, pan-fried ....
8	nonbreaded, pan-fried ....
7	roasted..
	liver

*See entry in Notes section for this class of food.

COMMON PORTION

AMOUNT	CSI	TOTAL CALORIES	TOTAL FAT GRAMS
4 oz.	7	185	4
4 oz.	8	260	16
4 oz.	5	145	6
4 oz.	5	169	8
5-inch	5	229	19
4 oz.	9	235	8
4 oz.	9	194	9
2 oz.	6	105	4
2 oz.	23	92	3
4 oz.	11	213	5
4 oz.	10	229	6
4 oz.	8	233	7
4 oz.	8	207	5
4 oz.	7	170	4

CSI	
	*veal (cont.)
35	braised...
24	pan-fried ....
	loin
10	braised...
9	roasted...
	rib
11	braised...
9	roasted...
10	shoulder, arm, braised ....
9	shoulder, arm, roasted ....
	shoulder, blade
11	braised...
10	roasted...
8	sirloin, braised..
8	sirloin, roasted..
	vegetable (see footnote 3, page 17)
	avocado, raw
3	California..
2	Florida ....
	beans
	baked
3	canned with franks ....
1	canned with pork....................................
3	home-prepared with pork......................

*See entry in Notes section for this class of food.

COMMON PORTION

AMOUNT	CSI	TOTAL CALORIES	TOTAL FAT GRAMS
4 oz.	35	186	8
4 oz.	24	277	13
4 oz.	10	255	10
4 oz.	9	198	8
4 oz.	11	246	9
4 oz.	9	201	8
4 oz.	10	227	6
4 oz.	9	185	7
4 oz.	11	223	7
4 oz.	10	194	8
4 oz.	8	230	7
4 oz.	8	190	7
1 medium	4	306	30
1 medium	5	339	27
½ cup	3	182	8
½ cup	1	133	2
½ cup	3	190	6

vegetable (cont.)

    refried

1   canned..

6   typical restaurant...................................

    broccoli, quiche

5   no egg yolk, milk 2% fat, typical crust ..

16   typical...

    cabbage roll (see cabbage roll)

5   eggplant Parmesan, typical...........................

    onion, rings

10   breaded, pan-fried in vegetable oil...........

10   pan-fried in vegetable oil by mfg., oven-
            heated...

    potato (white)

0   baked, with skin...

8   au gratin (whole milk 30%, cheddar
            cheese 9%, butter 3%) ....

7   au gratin (whole milk 30%, cheddar
            cheese 9%, margarine 3%)............

       chips (see chips)

2   baked, cheese-stuffed.................................

       French-fried

4   cottage-cut, pan-fried, oven-heated.......

6   frozen, restaurant deep-fried vegetable
              oil...

COMMON PORTION

AMOUNT	CSI	TOTAL CALORIES	TOTAL FAT GRAMS
½ cup	1	124	2
½ cup	6	243	14
4 oz.	5	327	21
6 oz.	24	480	38
1 cup	10	344	24
8 rings	7	275	16
8 rings	7	324	21
one 7 oz.	0	220	0
½ cup	9	160	9
½ cup	8	160	9
1 potato	4	236	10
10 strips	2	109	4
10 strips	3	158	8

vegetable (cont.)

5	frozen, pan-fried at home in vegetable oil ....
8	hash brown, homemade in vegetable oil .
	mashed
0	made with whole milk 15%, no butter or margarine ....
2	made with whole milk and butter........
1	made with whole milk and margarine .
	pancakes (see pancakes, potato)
	scalloped
3	made with whole milk 36%, butter 2%.
3	made with whole milk 36%, margarine 2%..
10	sticks...
	sweet (see vegetable, sweet potato)
	rice (see rice)
14	spinach, soufflé (cheddar cheese 13%, egg yolk 7%, butter 7%)...........................
	sweet potato
	(see footnote 3, page 17)
2	candied (butter 4%) ....
	taro, chips (see chips)
	zucchini
4	pie...

COMMON PORTION

AMOUNT	CSI	TOTAL CALORIES	TOTAL FAT GRAMS
10 strips	2	111	4
½ cup	5	151	9
½ cup	0	81	1
½ cup	2	111	4
½ cup	1	118	6
½ cup	4	105	4
½ cup	3	105	4
½ cup	2	94	6
1 cup	16	218	18
4 oz.	2	155	4
4 oz.	4	147	5

vegetable (cont.)
    casserole (see casserole)

8   **venison**, roasted ....

-W,Y-

wafers (see cookies)
waffles
2   made with oil, no egg yolks, skim milk .....
8   typical ....
2 **wheat germ**, toasted ....
whipped cream (see cream, whipped)
whipped imitation cream (cream, whipped)
yogurt
0   skim, dry nonfat milk added ....
2   low-fat, dry nonfat milk added....................
0   nonfat, frozen...
3   whole milk ....
4   cream added, frozen ....

-Z-

ziti (see footnote 3, page 17)

COMMON PORTION

AMOUNT	CSI	TOTAL CALORIES	TOTAL FAT GRAMS
4 oz.	8	178	4
one 7-inch	2	192	8
1 7-inch	8	249	13
1 tblsp.	0	27	1
1 cup	1	127	0
1 cup	3	144	4
1 cup	0	224	0
1 cup	6	139	7
1 cup	6	240	7

Notes

SPECIAL NOTES ON GROUPS OF FOODS

The following notes are in alphabetical order.

BEEF

Names of retail cuts of meat vary in different parts of the country. The U.S. Department of Agriculture listings we use are generic, without the imaginative names some stores give their meats. You may need the local butcher's help to relate local meat names to our USDA listings.

"Ribs 6–9," and "ribs 6–12" refer to the cuts of beef associated with those ribs. Butchers number the ribs from the front to the back of the animal. Although it is usual for patrons to refer to names like "top round," "bottom round," "prime ribs," etc., they may ask for cuts by rib numbers.

We list only *lean* cuts on the assumption that anyone interested in a low blood cholesterol level will want to eat only lean meat. Trim fat from meats before cooking.

Where possible, we list only those cuts trimmed to the least surface fat. Sometimes, however, the only figures that exist are for a cut trimmed no closer than ¼ inch of fat. We make clear which cuts these are.

Fat within meat fibers cannot be trimmed away. Often referred to as "marbling," it determines the grading of lean meat.

From least marbling to most marbling, the grades are: select, choice, prime.

CANDY

Hard candy, jelly beans, licorice, plain mints (no chocolate), taffy, marshmallows—all have zero or negligible CSIs when eaten in moderate amounts.

Carob is a chocolate substitute with a CSI of zero. Note it has approximately the same number of calories as chocolate.

CHICKEN

All figures are for meat only, no bones.

All figures for broilers also apply to fryers.

All listings assume cooked with or without the skin but always eaten *without* the skin. Eating the skin can raise the CSI for some pieces by almost 50 percent.

Beware of fast-food chicken coatings or any deep-fried chicken, which can double the CSI.

FISH

Many fish entries are listed as raw instead of cooked because no figures are available for cooked versions. Moist cooking would cause little change in the raw figures.

The flesh of all finfish contains *omega-3 fatty acids* that have shown evidence of lowering human blood total cholesterol and discouraging the formation of blood clots within arteries.

There is no way at present to quantify these two effects on the CSI. We can't say, for example, that you can cut the effective CSI number by 30 percent because of the beneficial consequences of omega-3 fatty acids. But we feel justified in saying that a higher CSI for some fish (e.g., Atlantic mackerel and Pacific herring) is offset to some extent by the omega-3 fatty acids.

Some dietary authorities recommend that you eat fish at least twice a week because of the omega-3 fatty acids.

HAM

Assume lean unless we specify "extra lean."

LAMB

We list only lean cuts. Within "lean," the USDA usually restricts itself to one grade, "choice."

All lamb is domestic unless specified as coming from New Zealand.

MARGARINE

To be legally called "margarine," a spread must contain a minimum of 80% fat. Spreads containing lesser amounts of fat are referred to in the marketplace as a "spread." They tend to have the lowest CSI value.

The CSI for a tablespoon of margarine or margarine-like spreads is the same as the saturated fat number listed in the package contents. If the saturated fat for one tablespoon is 2 grams, the CSI for a tablespoon would equal 2.

Most of the stick margarines have 2 grams of saturated fat per tablespoon. An exception is margarines made from safflower oil (e.g., Promise brand); they have only 1 gram of saturated fat per tablespoon and thus a CSI of 1.

To make margarine or margarine-like spreads, manufacturers add hydrogen to vegetable oil, a process called "hydrogenation." The more hydrogen you add

a) the stiffer the margarine or spread
b) the more saturated fat created.

Hydrogenation also creates a form of fatty acid called *trans* fatty acid. Recent studies show that these trans fatty acids can raise the blood cholesterol level.

Check the list of contents of the softer margarine-like spreads, especially the diet soft spreads. They tend to have the least saturated fat (therefore the lowest CSI) and the least amount of the trans fatty acids.

As to a choice between margarine and butter, compare:

1 tablespoon of margarine or spread CSI = 1 to 2
1 tablespoon of butter CSI = 9

Stay away from butter!

MAYONNAISE (see SALAD DRESSING)

OIL

Be careful when buying products advertised as "made with pure vegetable oil." "Vegetable oil" can include *tropical oils* (palm, coconut, palm kernel). Unlike vegetable oil made from corn, olives, soybeans, etc., the tropical oils are high in saturated fat and have a high CSI.

PASTA

All pastas can be made with or without eggs. Those without eggs will have a CSI = 0. Those with eggs can have a significant CSI that will be about the same for each shape of pasta (spaghetti, rigatoni, fettucini, etc.) but can have a different CSI depending on the manufacturer or restaurant chef. Check boxes when you buy. In the better restaurants, assume that the pasta contains eggs.

Few popular *pasta preparations* have been evaluated for saturated fat or cholesterol, and therefore few pasta preparations are listed. Two *pasta sauces* appear under "Sauce": marinara and canned spaghetti sauce.

POLYUNSATURATED FATS IN FOOD OILS AND FOOD OIL PRODUCTS

Oils and fats are molecules made up of long chains of carbon atoms that have hydrogen atoms attached. The greater the number of hydrogen atoms packed into each oil or fat molecule, the more it is "saturated" with hydrogen.

Some oils, such as canola oil and safflower oil, occur in nature relatively unsaturated; their molecules still have room for many more hydrogen atoms. The more food chemists pack them with hydrogen (a process called "hydrogenation"), the thicker these oils become until they start to stiffen into fat. This is how manufacturers make margarines from oils such as corn oil and canola oil.

The more an oil or fat is stiffened by this process, the more saturated fat it contains, and thus the higher its CSI number. In general, soft tub margarine has fewer hydrogen atoms, and thus a lower CSI, than does stick margarine. However, always check the label for the amount of saturated fat per tablespoon (preferably only one gram).

Polyunsaturated fat means fat with many places on the molecule still open to adding a hydrogen atom. Vegetable oils and the margarines made from them typically contain polyunsaturated fats. Authorities once thought that a large amount of polyunsaturated fat in the diet was beneficial. Now we know that there are problems with too much polyunsaturated fat: It tends to lower the blood concentration of the "good cholesterol," the HDL (high-density lipoprotein) fraction.

Today we say eat margarine instead of butter, but

with restraint. Use any oil or fat sparingly, of course, if only to avoid gaining weight.

PORK

With the exception of spareribs, only lean cuts appear.

PUDDINGS, DESSERT TYPE

All are made with whole milk unless otherwise stated.

SALAD, CHEF'S

The chef's salad figures are for a large salad (approximately 16 ounces) that you might get at dinner. Luncheon salads may be much smaller.

SALAD DRESSING, MAYONNAISE, "LOW-CALORIE" OR "IMITATION"

Check the package contents. Look for only 1 gram of saturated fat per tablespoon (14 grams).

SHELLFISH

All entries for clams are for mixed species.
While the flesh of all seafood contains *omega-3 fatty acids* that may lower human blood cholesterol and dis-

courage the formation of blood clots within the arteries, the amount in shellfish, shrimp, and lobster is too small to have a significant effect. Be guided by the CSI.

SOUPS

All soups are canned unless stated otherwise.
No figures are available for dehydrated soups reconstituted with milk.

SUNDAE DESSERTS

All are 5½-ounce by weight.

TURKEY

All figures are for meat only, no bones.
All figures for broilers also apply to fryers.
All listings assume cooked with or without the skin but always eaten *without* the skin. Eating the skin can raise the CSI for some pieces by almost 50 percent.

VEAL

We list only *lean* cuts of veal. The USDA does not differentiate grades (select, choice, etc.) for lean veal as it does for lean beef.

High CSI Food Groups

These food groups tend to have high CSI numbers:

organ meats: brains
gizzards
heart
intestines
kidneys
lungs
pancreas
sweetbreads (thymus)

tropical oils: coconut
palm
palm kernel

most cheeses (except special low-fat cheeses)

sausage, salami, regular bacon, bologna

butter, whole eggs, and egg yolks

prime cuts of beef, pork, lamb
spareribs
patés

pastry, including croissants

ice creams other than special low calorie or
fat-free

APPENDIX

DESIRABLE WEIGHT IN POUNDS*
(without shoes or clothes)

MEN

height in feet and inches	19–34 years of age	35 years and over
5' 0"	112–128	123–138
1"	116–132	127–143
2"	121–137	132–148
3"	124–141	136–152
4"	129–146	140–157
5"	132–150	144–162
6"	137–155	149–167
7"	141–160	153–172
8"	145–164	158–178
9"	149–169	163–183
10"	153–174	167–188
11"	158–179	173–194
6' 0"	162–184	177–199
1"	167–189	182–205
2"	172–195	187–210
3"	176–200	192–216
4"	181–205	198–222
5"	186–211	203–228
6"	190–216	208–234

Example: A 5'9", 64-year-old *man* should expect to weigh between 163 lbs. and 183 lbs.

WOMEN

height in feet and inches	19–34 years of age	35 years and over
5′ 0″	97–112	108–123
1″	101–116	111–127
2″	104–121	115–132
3″	107–124	119–136
4″	111–129	122–140
5″	114–132	126–144
6″	118–137	130–149
7″	121–141	134–153
8″	125–145	138–158
9″	129–149	142–163
10″	132–153	146–167
11″	136–158	151–173
6′ 0″	140–162	155–177
1″	144–167	159–182
2″	148–172	164–187
3″	152–176	168–192
4″	156–181	173–198

Example: A 5′9″, 64-year-old *woman* should expect to weigh between 142 lbs. and 163 lbs.

*Weight tables adapted from *Dietary Guidelines for Americans* (USDA and DHHS), 3rd ed., 1990

RECOMMENDED AVERAGE CALORIC INTAKE TO MAINTAIN WEIGHT*
FOR 20–39 YEARS OF AGE
(persons over 39 years of age please see below)

MEN

lbs.	little activity	mild activity	moderate activity	strenuous activity
90	1450	1650	1850	2200
100	1600	1800	2100	2450
110	1750	2000	2300	2700
120	1900	2200	2500	2900
130	2050	2350	2700	3150
140	2250	2550	2900	3400
150	2400	2700	3100	3650
160	2550	2900	3300	3900
170	2700	3100	3550	4150
180	2850	3250	3750	4400
190	3000	3450	3950	4650
200	3200	3600	4150	4850
210	3350	3800	4350	5100
220	3500	4000	4550	5350
230	3650	4150	4800	5600

*(See footnotes bottom of table for women on the next page and instructions top of page 166.)

WOMEN

lbs.	little activity	mild activity	moderate activity	strenuous activity
90	1400	1550	1650	1900
100	1550	1700	1800	2100
110	1700	1850	2000	2300
120	1850	2050	2150	2500
130	2000	2200	2350	2750
140	2150	2400	2550	2950
150	2300	2550	2700	3150
160	2450	2700	2900	3350
170	2600	2900	3100	3550
180	2750	3050	3250	3800
190	2900	3250	3450	4000
200	3050	3400	3600	4200
210	3200	3550	3800	4400
220	3350	3750	4000	4600
230	3500	3900	4150	4850

*Source: National Research Council (U.S.) Subcommittee of the 10th Ed. of the RDAs, National Academy of Sciences, 1989.

To adjust for over 39 years of age:
    40–49 years, multiply by 0.95
    50–59 years, multiply by 0.90
    60–69 years, multiply by 0.80
    70+ years, multiply by 0.70

(See example next page.)

Example: 160 lb., moderately active 64-year-old woman:

Go down the left column to 160 lbs. in the table for women and across that 160-lb. row to the column marked "moderate activity" to find the figure 2,900 calories.

Because this woman is between 60 and 69 years old, multiply 2,900 by 0.8 = *2,320 calories*. This is the recommended caloric intake to maintain her 160-lb. weight.

Examples of levels of activity:

mild activity:	cleaning house
	office work
	baseball
	golf
moderate activity:	brisk walk (3-4 mph)
	gardening
	cycling (5 mph)
	dancing
	basketball
strenuous activity:	jogging (9 mph)
	football
	swimming

Most people underestimate the calories they eat by as much as 25 to 40 percent. People who report 2,000 calories often actually consume as much as 3,000 calories. You really need to keep track of calories by carefully recording the amount of food you eat and its method of preparation. A dietitian can help if you find estimating calories difficult to do on your own.

Persons who have undergone significant weight loss and weight gain by dieting usually have an altered metabolism. It can make this table inaccurate for them. They definitely should consult a professional.

RECOMMENDED DAILY TOTAL CSI TARGET

calories per day	CSI for mild fat restriction (30%)	CSI for moderate fat restriction (25%)	CSI for strict fat restriction (20%)
1200	19	17	10
1400	22	20	12
1600	25	23	13
1800	28	26	15
2000	32	28	17
2200	34	31	18
2400	38	34	20
2600	41	37	22
2800	44	40	23
3000	47	43	25
3200	51	45	27
3400	53	48	28
3600	57	51	30
3800	60	54	32
4000	63	57	33

[Adapted from "The New American Diet"—see reference on page 184.]

Using this table:

After you have determined the proper daily calories for your weight using the previous tables, find the CSI for the level of fat restriction you want to achieve.

Example:

We have determined in a previous example that a 64-year-old moderately active woman needs about *2,320* calories. That would put her approximately halfway between the 2,200 and 2,400 levels in the first column of this table. Her 30 percent fat restriction CSI target would then be *36* (halfway between 34 and 38 in column 2).

Once you achieve the 30 percent-fat-restriction CSI level, you may want to attempt a 25 percent level. In the example of the 64-year-old woman, that would be between 31 and 34 (column 3 above).

The really ambitious can try for the most benefit, the 20 percent restriction. Just remember to give yourself lots of time. And certainly give yourself credit for whichever of the three levels you achieve!

ADJUSTING FOR YOUR "USUAL PORTION"

If your *usual portion* of any food differs from the *common portion* in the table, you can easily calculate the CSI, calories, or total fat for your *usual* portion. The examples below are CSI calculations.

Procedure:
1. Divide *your usual portion* by the *book common portion*.
2. Multiply the result by the book *CSI* value.

Example 1:
Your usual portion of corned beef is 6 ounces. The *book common portion* for corned beef is 4 ounces.

1. Divide:

$$\frac{\text{usual portion}}{\text{book common portion}} \quad \frac{6 \text{ oz.}}{4 \text{ oz.}}$$
= 1.5, which is the *multiplier*.

2. Multiply:
   1.5 × the *book CSI* for corned beef of 13 = 19.5

which we would round off to *20*. This is the CSI for your *usual portion*.

Example 2: Suppose you eat only 3 ounces of corned beef.
As shown above,

1. Divide *your usual portion* by the book *common portion*:

$$\frac{\text{your usual portion}}{\text{book common portion}} \quad \frac{3 \text{ oz.}}{4 \text{ oz.}}$$

which equals 0.75 (the *multiplier*).

2. Therefore, multiply

$$0.75 \times \text{corned beef CSI of } 13 = 9.7$$

which we would round off to *10*. This is your *usual portion* CSI for corned beef.

Note: The multiplier is also used to adjust for your usual portion of total fat or calories.

> In *example 1* we calculated a multiplier of 1.5 for a 6-ounce usual portion. Consulting the book table, we see that the common 4-ounce portion of corned beef has

$$\text{total fat} = 21 \text{ gms.}$$
$$\text{calories} = 283$$

Multiply each of these by 1.5 to get the values for your 6-ounce usual portion:

$$\text{total fat} = 21 \times 1.5 = 32 \text{ gms.}$$
$$\text{calories} = 283 \times 1.5 = 425 \text{ calories}$$

OPTIONAL CALCULATIONS

The following examples allow you to

1. calculate the CSI yourself
2. calculate your total fat intake

1. CALCULATING THE CSI YOURSELF

You can calculate the CSI if you know the *grams (gms.) of saturated fat* and the *milligrams (mgs.) of cholesterol* for a particular weight or volume of a product. The formula is

$$CSI = 1.01 \times gms. \text{ of saturated fat} + 0.05 \times mg. \text{ of cholesterol}$$

Example:
Most margarines have the saturated fat and cholesterol contents on their labels. One tablespoon (14 grams) of a product might contain *2 grams* of saturated fat and *0 milligrams* of cholesterol:

$$CSI = 1.01 \times 2 + 0.05 \times 0 = 2.02$$

which we would round off to 2.

Remember, though, that this CSI = 2 is for one tablespoon (14 grams or ½ ounce), which is probably the average amount you put on a slice of bread. Put it on twice as thick and you double the CSI to 4.

Note: It really makes no practical difference whether you multiply the grams of fat by 1.01 or by 1. However, the official formula is 1.01.

2. CALCULATIONS FOR TOTAL FAT

Two questions are of immediate interest for those who want to limit the total fat in their diet:

A. I know the number of calories I consume on an average day. What percentage of those calories is coming from the fat in the foods I eat?

B. Now I want to set a limit on calories from fat to less than 30 percent of my total calories. What is the number of calories that would be less than 30 percent of my total calories?

A. Calculating the Percentage of Calories in Your Diet That Comes From Fat

You have added up the grams of fat consumed in a day. You want to know if the calories coming from that fat exceed 30 percent.

Basic fact: Each gram of fat eaten supplies 9 calories.

Example:
   your total calories = 2,100 for the day
   your total fat = 72 gms. for the day

1. Multiply 72 gms. of fat × 9 = *648 calories from fat*
2. *650 calories from fat* divided by *2,100 total calories* = 0.309.

3. To convert to percent, multiply 0.309 by 100 = 30.9 percent, which we would round off to 31 percent.

Therefore, if you consumed 2,100 total calories and 72 grams of fat in a day, 31 percent of your calories came from fat.

(Since we do not list most foods from groups such as fruit, grain, etc., with CSIs of zero, find their calories in one of the reference works we have cited on page 184.)

B. Calculating the Number of Calories From Fat To Be Less Than 30 Percent

You know the number of calories you consume in a day and want to know the maximum number of those calories that can come from fat without exceeding 30 percent of calories from fat.

We will use the 30 percent level for our example.

Example: You average 2,500 calories a day.

Multiply 0.30 (representing 30 percent) by 2,500 calories = *750 calories*.

You now know that no more than 750 calories can come from fat or you will exceed the 30 percent limit.

(For a 25 percent or 20 percent limit on calories from fat, substitute 0.25 for 25 percent or 0.20 for 20 percent in the formula.)

Recipe Substitutes for Low CSI Cooking

Recipe Original	Recipe Substitute
butter	vegetable oil margarine or margarine-like spreads (but no palm or coconut oil)* canola oil in baking (not frying)* vegetable oil spray in cooking* powdered butter substitutes (e.g., "Molly McButter," "Butter Buds," etc.)
eggs	3 egg whites for 2 whole eggs 2 tablsp. of commercial egg substitutes for each whole egg, especially baking ("Scramblers," "Egg Beaters," etc.)
ham	turkey ham (this is processed turkey that resembles ham)

*Be aware that these substitutes contain the same number of calories as the products they replace.

french fries	oven-baked "fries"
cream cheese	Neufchatel cheese, light cream cheese
whole milk	skim milk
cream	nondairy creamer (without coconut oil!)* evaporated milk*
sour cream	nonfat plain yogurt
cheese	low-fat cheese (less than 5 gms. of fat per ounce); if for melting, 5 to 6 gms. of fat per oz.
mayonnaise	low-fat or fat-free mayonnaise (5 gms. of total fat and 1 gm. of saturated fat per tablsp.)
salad dressing	low-fat or fat-free salad dressings
ground meat	10 percent fat ground meat (beef or poultry)
oil for sautéing	vegetable oil spray
for marinating	low-fat or fat-free salad dressings

*Be aware that these substitutes contain the same number of calories as the products they replace.

baking flour	cake flour has less gluten, yields a more tender product*
wok oil	stir fry in broth or wine
fat in baking	fruit pulp or purée for moistness and smoothness
	nonfat or low-fat yogurt (acidic) to replace some or all fat
fat in frying	use a nonstick pan
thickening sauces	cooked potato or onion purée
cake	angel-food cake; fat-free commercial cakes

For a large number of low-CSI recipes, see *The New American Diet System* at the end of the Notes section of this book, page 184.

*Be aware that these substitutes contain the same number of calories as the products they replace.

Sample Low-CSI Meals

BREAKFAST

	AMOUNT	CSI	GMS. OF FAT
fruit (any)	1 medium	0	0
oatmeal	⅔ cup	0	2
cocoa with skim milk	1 cup	0	2
totals		0	4
fruit (any)	1 medium	0	0
dry cereal*	¾ cup	0	0
plus skim milk	½ cup	0	0
cocoa (skim milk)	1 cup	2	2
totals		2	2

*No coconut, nuts, or oil

177

	AMOUNT	CSI	GMS. OF FAT
fruit (any)	1 medium	0	0
rye toast with tub margarine-like	3 slices	0	0
spread	2 tblsp.	2	14
coffee	1 cup	0	0
milk, 2%	2 tblsp.	1	1
totals		3	15
fruit (any)	1 medium	0	0
French toast, made with egg substitute, skim milk	2 slices	2	8
Canadian bacon	1 oz.	2	3
coffee with	1 cup	0	0
milk, 2%	2 tblsp.	1	1
totals		5	12
fruit (any)	1 medium	0	0
egg white omelet with tub margarine-like	3 whites	0	0
spread	1 tblsp.	1	7
pumpernickel toast with margarine (corn oil, tub)	2 slices	0	2
	2 tblsp.	2	14
coffee with	1 cup	0	0
milk, 2%	2 tblsp.	1	1
totals		4	24

LUNCH

	AMOUNT	CSI	GMS. OF FAT
soup, chicken noodle with meatballs, ready to serve	1 cup	1	4
pita	1 pocket	0	1
cheese, Dorman's light	2 oz.	1	10
lettuce, tomato, sprouts	½ cup	0	0
fruit, any	1 medium	0	0
totals		2	15
salad, large tossed	2 cups	0	0
olive oil	1 tblsp.	2	14
vinegar	1 tblsp.	0	0
chili with chicken and beans	1 cup	1	4
soda crackers, regular	6	1	2
totals		4	20
sandwich:			
rye bread	2 slices	0	0
ham roast, extra lean, canned	4 oz.	4	6
mustard	1 tblsp.	0	0
fruit (any)	1 medium	0	0
totals		4	6

	AMOUNT	CSI	GMS. OF FAT
soup, black bean, condensed, water prepared	1 cup	0	2
sandwich:			
French bread	2 slices	0	1
turkey, white meat	4 oz.	5	4
light mayonnaise	1 tblsp.	1	5
fruit (any)	1 medium	0	0
totals		6	12
sandwich:			
Italian bread	2 slices	0	0
chicken, light meat, roasted	4 oz.	6	5
lettuce and tomato	½ cup	0	0
light mayonnaise	1 tblsp.	1	5
gingersnap cookies	1 oz.	2	3
totals		9	13
hamburger (10% fat)	4 oz.	9	9
French fries, small	10 strips	3	8
diet or regular soft drink	12 oz.	0	0
totals		12	17

DINNER

	AMOUNT	CSI	GMS. OF FAT
trout, rainbow, broiled	4 oz.	5	5
with lemon	⅛ oz.	0	0
wild rice mix with	1 cup	0	0
tub margarine-like			
spread	1 tblsp.	1	7
roll	1 oz.	0	0
green beans with steamed			
mushrooms	½ cup	0	0
fruit, mixed fresh	1 cup	0	0
totals		6	12
chicken, light meat,			
roasted	4 oz.	6	5
potato, baked, with	1 lrge.	0	0
tub margarine-like			
spread	1 tblsp.	1	7
carrots, steamed with			
parsley	½ cup	0	0
lettuce and tomato salad,	1 cup	0	0
with Russian			
dressing	2 tblsp.	1	6
angelfood cake with fruit	⅒ cake	0	0
totals..................................		8	18

	AMOUNT	CSI	GMS. OF FAT
chowder, Manhattan clam	1 cup	1	3
beef, eye of round, broiled	4 oz.	6	5
sweet potato, baked, with margarine (corn oil, tub)	1 medium	0	0
	1 tablsp.	1	7
spinach, steamed, with lemon	1 cup	0	0
frozen yogurt, nonfat	1 cup	0	0
totals		8	15
Spaghetti (no egg)	8 oz.	0	0
Italian meat sauce	½ cups	6	10
Italian bread with tub margarine-like	2 big slices	0	0
spread	1 tblsp.	1	7
salad, tossed with	2 cups	0	0
olive oil	1 tblsp.	2	14
vinegar	1 tblsp.	0	0
totals		9	31

RESTAURANT MEAL

	AMOUNT	CSI	GMS. OF FAT
grouper, broiled	6 oz.	5	2
potato, baked	1 lrge.	0	0
with light sour cream	2 tblsp.	5	6
vegetable, steamed	½ cup	0	0
salad with	2 cups	0	0
olive oil	1 tblsp.	2	14
vinegar	1 tblsp.	0	0
bread,	1 oz.	0	0
with butter	2 pats	4	8
sorbet	1 cup	0	0
mints	handful	0	1
coffee	1 cup	0	0
with cream (half-and-half)	1 tblsp.	2	2
totals		18	33

Sources

We derived our figures from

United States Department of Agriculture (USDA) handbooks, "Composition of Foods"

Food Values of Portions Commonly Used, Pennington, J. A., Harper & Row, New York, 15th ed., 1989

The New American Diet System, Connor, S. L., and Connor, W. E., Simon & Schuster, New York, 1991
  (The two authors of this reference led the research team that created the CSI formula. Their large book contains an extensive section of valuable low-CSI recipes.)

Food Values: Cholesterol and Fats, Wallach, Leah, Perennial Library, Harper & Row, New York, 1989

Nutritionist III, Version 7.2 Computer Program N-Squared Computing, Salem, OR

Your Suggestions for This Book

Do you have ideas to improve this book?

What favorite foods (other than commercial preparations) do you wish we had included?

We will give careful consideration to your suggestions for the next edition. If we use your suggestion, we'll gladly send you a free copy of the new edition.

Please write to

Explanatory Publications
70 Kenilworth Drive East
Stamford, CT 06902

or Fax 203-325-2464

Thank you!

About the Authors

JOEL M. BERNS, D.M.D., a diplomate of the American Board of Oral Surgery, is a retired oral surgeon who has been interested in the cholesterol question for a number of years because of his own experience following a low-cholesterol diet. He is the owner and editor in chief of Explanatory Publications, a company creating works explaining medical and dental subjects to the laity.

Consultant KENNETH L. COHEN, M.D., F.A.C.P., a diplomate of the American Board of Internal Medicine and certified in the subspecialty of endocrinology and metabolism, is an associate professor of medicine, Section of Medicine and Endocrinology, Yale-New Haven Hospital, and associate chief of staff for ambulatory care at the Veterans Administration Medical Center, West Haven, CT. He lectures extensively on lipid disorders for the Yale Affiliated Hospital Program and oversees the Metabolic Clinic at the West Haven VA Hospital. He is a member of the core faculty of the Cardiac Preventive Health Program at Yale University.

Consultant BETSY A. TAYLOR, M.S., R.D., is the program director for Health Extenders, a health-risk reduction medical practice in Norwalk, CT, where she treats patients with dietary problems for control of obesity, cardiac disease, and diabetes. She was until recently chief clinical dietitian at the Hampton General Hospital, Hampton, VA, and before that a research assistant at the United States Department of Agriculture in Beltsville, MD. She has been a guest lecturer at the Yale University School of Medicine.